A DOCTOR'S PRESCRIPTION

A DOCTOR'S PRESCRIPTION

For Getting the Best Medical Care

KURT LINK, M.D.

DEMBNER BOOKS • New York

Dembner Books
Published by Red Dembner Enterprises Corp.,
80 Eighth Avenue, New York, N.Y. 10011
Distributed by W. W. Norton & Company, Inc.,
500 Fifth Avenue, New York, N.Y. 10110

Copyright © 1990 by Kurt Link, M.D.

All rights reserved. No part of this book may be reproduced in any form without permission in writing from the publisher, except by a reviewer who wishes to quote brief passages in connection with a review written for inclusion in a magazine, newspaper, or broadcast. Printed in the United States of America.

Library of Congress Cataloging-in-Publication Data

Link, Kurt, 1937–
    A doctor's prescription for getting the best medical care / Kurt Link.
      p. cm.
    Includes index.
    ISBN 0-942637-15-1 : $19.95
    1. Medicine, Popular. 2. Health. 3. Consumer education.
I. Title. II. Title: Doctor's prescription for getting the best
medical care. III. Title: Doctor's Rx. IV. Title: Doctor's
prescription.
RC81.L645   1990   89-30969
610—dc19   CIP

Design by Antler & Baldwin, Inc.

TO JUDY

CONTENTS

Introduction   1

1. **Choosing the Right Doctor** *by Kurt Link, M.D.*   5
   Generalist or Specialist, 5
   The Good Doctor, 8
   Recognized Medical Boards, 17

2. **Choosing a Health Insurance** *by Kurt Link, M.D.*   26
   How It All Got Started, 26
   Health Insurance, 29
   HMO—Health Maintenance Organizations, 33
   PPO—Preferred Provider Organizations, 41
   Medicare, 44
   Medicaid, 48
   Choosing a Medical Insurance Plan, 49

3. **Medical Tests** *by Kurt Link, M.D.*   54
   Selecting and Interpreting Tests, 54
   Why Test and When? 59
   Commonly Used Tests, 61
   Disorders and Solutions, 71

4. **Medications** *by Kurt Link, M.D.*   75
   The Risks, 76
   The Benefits, 84
   Commonly Used Medications, 91
   The Cost Factor and the Use of Generics, 100

5. **Surgery** *by Kurt Link, M.D.*   105
   History of Surgery, 105
   Risk–Benefit Ratio, 112

Risks, 115
Benefits, 128
Surgical Techniques, 129
Kinds of Surgery, 131

6. **Substance Abuse** *by Marigail Wynne, M.D.*   137
   Dependency Substances, 139
   Addiction, Abuse, and Dependence, 145
   Causes of Addiction, 147
   Treatment, 148
   The Family Illness of Chemical Dependency, 150

7. **Nutrition** *by Patricia Simko-Imhof, R.D.*   153
   Understanding the Basics, 154
   Obesity: Theories and Myths, 169
   What Is a Nutritionist? 175
   Nutrition in Perspective, 178

8. **Staying Healthy** *by Kurt Link, M.D.*   180
   Life-Style, 180
   Immunizations, 184
   The Periodic Checkup, 185

9. **Medical Malpractice** *by Carolyn LaVecchia, R.N., F.N.P., M.S., J.D.*   188
   What Is Medical Malpractice? 189
   Types of Medical Malpractice Cases, 194
   Is There a Case? 196
   Insurance Crisis or Medical Malpractice Crisis? 201

Bibliography   203

Index   208

ACKNOWLEDGMENTS

My family put up with my many long disappearances into the attic/study, and spared me many a chore and many a carpool trip so that I could find the time to do this work. My colleagues Bob Goodman, Charlie Cook, Hank Stoneburner, and Jim Darden gave me the benefit of their time and particular expertise. Robin Wright thoughtfully reviewed much of the book. Aided by Karen Friloux, Priscilla Ronzitti's eagle eye and quiet discipline did much to shape the manuscript. My editor clarified, strengthened, and polished my prose, and showed me how to change the manuscript in important and constructive ways. My coauthors, pressed as they were by a thousand professional and personal responsibilities, came through on time. To all, my thanks and gratitude.

Kurt Link

INTRODUCTION

The capabilities of scientific medicine are awesome. Smallpox, a disfiguring and often fatal infection that terrified mankind since the fifteenth century, has recently been abolished from the earth. In developed countries the death of a child, an event that for centuries was a thing to be expected, to be taken for granted, is today seen as an unexpected tragedy. The agony of uremic poisoning can now be prevented by the artificial kidney machine. Even in the case of terminal heart failure, life and function can sometimes be preserved by a heart transplant. Individuals with injuries that once were always fatal now often survive and fully recover.

In spite of these great and continuing successes, there has been a growing disenchantment with modern scientific medicine. Malpractice litigation increases yearly; there is a whole library of books critical of doctors and medicine. The problems with modern medicine are not subtle or superficial; they are rooted in the very same scientific methods and thinking that are the source of medicine's triumphs.

Twentieth-century American medicine grew out of the dangerous, capricious, and irrational practices that characterized even the best medicine of the eighteenth and even most of the nineteenth century. Before the Civil War most medical training was based on the seventeenth century apprenticeship system.

Toward the end of the nineteenth century the apprenticeship was supplemented with formal education of several months in a medical school. The only requirement in the medical schools of the day was the ability to pay the tuition, which lined the pockets of the entrepreneurial physicians who owned and operated these proprietary schools. In approximately 100 years the United States and Canada produced 457 such medical schools. Although the education provided by these schools was inferior by modern standards, they had the virtue of having a heterogenous student body. Women, blacks, and the poor were well represented. Because of the great expense of providing high quality teaching in a medical school, many of these schools didn't last very long and neither did the diversity of the student body.

There were few available medications. Most therapies were at best harmless and often dangerous. The almost routine use of calomel to purge the body of various poisons or humors resulted in acute and chronic mercury poisoning, diarrhea, dehydration, and electrolyte depletion. The few medicines that had the potential for real therapeutic value, such as quinine (malaria), opium (pain), digitalis (heart failure), and colchicine (gout) were often prescribed for the wrong ailments, and so even these did more harm than good. The use of bleeding was encouraged by the famous physician, Benjamin Rush, who believed that the basis of all disease was physiologic tension, especially for the arteries and veins. He bled patients for any acute illness. Bleeding was practiced until 1870.(1)* George Washington's demise was surely hastened by this practice. Wiser men, such as Jacob Bigelow, who recognized that many patients get better without treatment(2), were unheeded.

Beginning in the eighteenth century, the more inquiring and ambitious minds, seeking a more intellectual and challenging education, traveled to the great hospitals and lecture halls of Europe. Returning from abroad, these individuals became the first teachers of scientific medicine. This new approach to healing had begun to emerge in the late seventeenth century, following the discovery of bacteria as the specific cause of some diseases. Until that discovery, disease was believed to be due to an imbalance of various forces or humors. But with the discovery of bacteria and the development of the germ theory of disease, the seminal concept of the existence of a specific cause for each specific disease was formulated. At the same time new and powerful specific therapies were emerging. Antitoxins and vaccinations led to further search for a "magic bullet" for every infection. There followed then the discovery of the causes of many of man's ancient pestilences, and then later the cause of diabetes, strokes, and many other medical afflictions. In the decades between 1920 and 1950 scientific medicine was perhaps in its most successful and popular phase. Those years saw the appearance of antibiotics, vaccinations, blood transfusions, and stunning new surgical successes. For the first time the victim of tuberculosis, blood poisoning, bacterial endocarditis, and pneumococcal pneumonia could be cured and the victim of major trauma and hemorrhage could survive.

The ensuing decades have seen incredible technological marvels that prolong life and relieve disability in ways not even dreamed of previously. But the science that made these advances possible encouraged a narrow view of the patient, and of health and disease. If a thing couldn't be measured or at

*Parenthetical numbers refer to entries in the Bibliography, pg. 203 ff.

least observed, it tended to be ignored. A disease was seen as the result of a noxious agent, a microbe for example, acting on a passive patient-host. Today we recognize illness as a dynamic interaction among the agent, the patient, and the environment. "Health" could too easily be defined as the absence of disease, or, even more narrowly, the condition in which all available tests and measurements are in a normal range. Sometimes the patient was examined like a biological specimen, without regard to his social context, physical environment, recuperative powers, or feelings. Osler and the other great physicians always recognized the importance of their patients' humanity, but lesser students often became so enthralled with the science that they forgot the person.

More recently the new technology and powerful new drugs have brought with them new problems. The ability to keep alive the desperately or hopelessly ill has not automatically brought with it the wisdom to know when to do so and when not to do so. Iatrogenic (caused by a physician or treatment) disease sometimes accompanies the use of hormones, antibiotics, and other drugs that affect the body's chemistry and organ function. We now see the so-called diseases of medical progress. These are diseases directly or indirectly caused by medical therapy. For example, patients can now be kept alive even when their illness is so severe and advanced that their natural defenses are almost wholly destroyed. As a result they develop infections never before seen, sometimes by what would ordinarily be harmless microbes. Other patients develop unheard of metabolic and chemical derangements that were previously incompatible with life.

An additional problem is the incredible expense of modern medicine, exacerbating the age-old problem of how to control costs and fairly distribute health care. New kinds of health insurance and payment methods are appearing in an attempt to address this issue, although no definitive solution is in sight.

Added to these problems is the common problem of poor doctor-patient communication, made somewhat worse by the historical and social forces that have dictated that, until recently, almost all American physicians were white middle- or upper-middle-class males, carrying their unavoidable biases and value systems.

Modern scientific medicine has at various times been accused of treating patients as objects, of ignoring the body's natural healing powers, of emphasizing sickness instead of health, and of ignoring preventive medicine. There is, unfortunately, some truth to all these charges. We physicians tend to be most comfortable with a patient who has a well-defined disease of known cause and for which there is an effective treatment. Life, however, does not come so neatly packaged. I think that the medical profession is starting to come to terms with that. Medical school curricula are devoting more time to communication skills, to ethical problems, and to consideration of the patient as a whole person, not just the repository of a disease. But problems remain, and you will have to deal with them when you seek medical care.

Medicine today can be powerful and effective, but to avoid the problems, and to get the best possible care you will have to make the right choices. I hope this book will help.

1

CHOOSING THE RIGHT DOCTOR
Kurt Link, MD

Finding a doctor who is right for you can be difficult for several reasons. For one thing, the information you need to make a logical choice is sometimes not available. But even if you do have that information and make a perfectly logical choice, that does not take into account the personality and practice style of the physician. If these are not also right for you, the choice may not be a good one.

Another problem is that there are sometimes limitations on the choices that you can make. There may be a limited number of physicians available in your community, you may not be able to afford the doctor of your choice, or your health insurance plan may limit you to physicians on a panel. This last concern is discussed in some detail in the chapter on health insurance.

But in any case, you will have choices available, so the question is: How are you to go about making the right one?

When I started out in practice, an older doctor told me that my success would depend on three things: my availability, affability, and ability—in that order. He may have been partly right. But those are not the only factors that determine a patient's choice of doctor.

GENERALIST OR SPECIALIST

The most obvious question to begin with is what kind of physician to choose: generalist or specialist? In a sense all physicians are specialists today. Gone is the old-fashioned GP. He is extinct, and for good reason. He was the man who started practice immediately after medical school, usually taking an apprenticeship, or else he started his own practice after a year's internship following medical school. He delivered babies, performed surgery (minor and often major), took care of infants, children, and adults. The specialist, by contrast, took a residency of two or more years after the internship *and* restricted his practice to one particular field. This worked reasonably well until the technology and complexity of medicine increased so dramatically in the 1950s and 1960s that training beyond the internship came to be seen as necessary for any practitioner. So the GP gave way to the new breed—the specialist in family practice.

Thus the modern choice is between primary-care clinician and specialist or, more likely, subspecialist.

Primary care does not belong to any one specialty. Primary care can be practiced by a family medicine specialist, an internist, a pediatrician, an obstetrician, or even a general surgeon. Whatever his training, his job is the same: to be available, to provide the initial examination and treatment or, when necessary, referral to a subspecialist. He is the one to see if you don't feel good and don't know what the matter is. He is the one to direct you to a subspecialist if you need one. He is supposed to know you as a person and not see you as a case. He is interested not only in finding disease but also in promoting health. He knows what maladies you, in particular, are at risk for, and makes his examinations and recommendations accordingly. He is interested in preventing you from getting sick, and to that end recommends vaccines and screening tests such as mammography, PAP smears, and tests of the stool for blood. He doesn't restrict his attention to the problem that is bothering you. He will check your blood pressure if you see him for a cold; he will detect your heart murmur even if you complain only about a stomach ulcer. His knowledge is broad, his concerns comprehensive. He strives to see the whole picture. If you have multiple medical problems, he is your best bet. If you have diabetes and high blood pressure and asthma, you may need more than one doctor, but there is one doctor you surely need—your primary-care physician. He will coordinate your treatments and resolve conflicting advice. He will minimize the numbers of visits and tests and tend to be conservative in his treatment.

Unfortunately, the primary care physician's virtues contain the key to his potential vices. At worst he may be busy, superficial, and ignorant. Any doctor may be too busy for his patients' good. This is especially likely to be true for the primary-care physician. Since he is on the front lines, it is harder for him to say no when called by a distressed patient, even if his schedule is already full. Economic factors also play a role. The primary-care physician's income is heavily dependent on the volume of his practice—unlike his subspecialty brethren whose relatively large fees for high-tech procedures and examinations allow, at least theoretically, a somewhat more leisurely pace.

The necessary breadth of the primary-care physician's practice means that his knowledge is of limited depth. "Keeping up" is difficult for all physicians, but especially for those who see a wide variety of cases. Indeed, one of the attractions of being a specialist or superspecialist (there are physicians who specialize in only one part of the eye, for example) is the confidence that comes with feeling truly expert. No matter how many journals he reads, conferences and meetings and lectures he attends, cassette tapes he hears, or consultations he requests, the practicing physician still knows that his knowledge is limited and perhaps already outdated. But if he has a keen awareness of his limitations, he can practice safe and effective medicine.

Consider, then, the specialist. His job is to know his stuff. He is the one to see if your case requires up-to-the-minute knowledge, familiarity with rare diseases or rare manifestations of common disease, or the application of the new high-technology medicine. He is the one who will, depending on his specialty, look directly into your bladder, colon, or bronchial tubes. He is the one who can measure the pressures in the heart chambers and arteries of the lungs; he can biopsy your liver, kidney, lungs, and even your heart or brain. If he is a surgical subspecialist, he has a professional lifetime of experience with the particular operation you need. He may do microsurgery with stitches so small that he has to use a microscope to see the suture material; or he may use laser beams to cut through tissue or repair the retina; or he may send a small, collapsed balloon to an otherwise unreachable artery and, by inflating it, widen a dangerously narrowed segment.

He must know what his techniques and procedures can do, and he must know when to use them. He must also know when not to use them. He must use, develop, and extend new technology. But he must also control and restrain it so that it is used in the service of your best interests. Sometimes the most difficult diagnosis to make is the absence of disease. You may have a symptom, or an abnormal medical test which suggests some (usually feared) disease such as heart disease, multiple sclerosis (MS), or hidden cancer. Proving that you do *not* have such an ailment may require all the professional and personal skills of the most highly trained specialist.

So why not consult a specialist (assuming you know what kind of specialist you need) every time you need a doctor? Like everyone else, the specialist tends to do what he knows how to do and recognize the familiar. The nephrologist is sure to look at your urine, the hematologist will look at your blood smear, the cardiologist will do an EKG, the lung specialist will do breathing tests, and the urologist will check your prostate. And each is likely to do tests that none of the others will. If you are suffering from hayfever, which can be treated with antihistamines and other medications or with allergy shots, it is the allergist who is more likely to choose the shots.

Some specialists make it clear that they will focus only on your problems within their field. Although this is a widely accepted practice, and tends to ensure that the care you receive from the specialist is up to date and competent, it can result in the neglect of other potentially important problems. Even if the specialist does take an interest in your other problems, he may prefer to refer you to another specialist for treatment. So, by going to a specialist, you may end up needing multiple physicians to care for your multiple problems. This can be costly and inconvenient, and at times compromise your medical care.

There are some other categories of medical care available, including a non-MD clinician such as the nurse practitioner and the physician's assistant. Most nurse practitioners were originally working RNs who decided to take the additional training in clinical medicine necessary to become certified and licensed as nurse practitioners. They frequently specialize in such areas as family medicine, obstetrics, pediatrics, or cardiology. Although they may be independent practitioners, they commonly work closely with a physician preceptor, especially in HMOs, large clinics, and teaching hospitals. You may be more comfortable with a nurse practitioner than a physician because she (or, less often, he) may be less intimidating, more interested in educating and communicating with you, and may have more time to spend with you. It is therefore no surprise that, in the right setting, the medical care provided by nurse practitioners compares favorably with that provided by physicians. Many patients who have had experience with both kinds of practitioners prefer the nurse practitioner.

Physician's assistants are not nurses; they pursue an independent study course that also leads to licensure. Physician's assistants (PAs) are not independent practitioners and tend to be used most for standarized, technical procedures—doing tests, suturing superficial wounds, making basic physical examination, and so on. They may have had previous experience as corpsmen, ambulance attendants, or other paramedical personnel. In some practice settings they may function much like a nurse practitioner.

With the exception of the rare nurse practitioner in an independent private practice, these nonphysician clinicians work with physicians. They are not a substitute for your doctor, but to his care they can add the dimension of greater accessibility, their own empathy, communication skills, and personality. If you have unmet needs in these areas, this may be the clinician for you.

THE GOOD DOCTOR

Let us assume that you have decided on what kind of doctor you want. The task now is to pick a good one. But how do you know if a doctor is "good"? Indeed, how do you even define "good"? An obvious way to define a good doctor is "one who gets his patients better"—his results are good. There are other ways: He can be compassionate, supportive; he can be a teacher or an inspiration; he can set an example. But in this discussion let us focus on his results: Does he help his patients? Is he better or worse at monitoring their health than the doctor down the road? Unfortunately, this information is not generally available. Doctors themselves do not know how they compare to other doctors in this regard. Some information from hospitals is available, thanks to Medicare, which has mandated PROs (Peer Review Organizations) to monitor the care of hospitalized Medicare patients. This is beginning to provide some information about individual physician's practices, but the data is not generally available to the public. Even if it were, it would be of little help in that it is geared to detection of deviant and inadequate care and detects only flagrant problems. Furthermore, knowing what percentage of a doctor's patients get better does not necessarily indicate his skill. A nationally known specialist who cares for the sickest patients may have a higher death rate than a lesser skilled practitioner, who sees many patients whose conditions get better by themselves.

This brings up another problem with this kind of evaluation of a doctor's performance. It is difficult to show that one physician is better than another because the outcome of illness for the majority of patients is not affected by what the doctor does. A large number of patients will get better regardless of treatment; some will die in spite of the best treatment; only a small number of patients' cure or survival will depend on the doctor.

Thus, this most rational way of picking a good doctor is not feasible because either the data is not available or, if available, almost uninterpretable. It may be helpful, however, to review five characteristics of your potential doctor: his education, training, and qualifications; his reputation; his experience; his availability; and his personality and practice style. If you can obtain information on these points, there is a good chance you will find a competent individual who will give you good service.

Education, Training, and Qualifications

Determining a doctor's education, training, and qualifications is probably the easiest. You can ask him or his office staff. This very direct approach may give you the information you seek and possibly other information as well. You may get a direct and adequate reply, evasiveness, or a downright refusal. You may find the doctor frankly forthcoming, defensive, suspicious, or even hostile. If you are dissatisfied with his response, you may have quickly determined that he is not the person for you. It is of course possible that an otherwise excellent physician can be touchy if you appear to be questioning his competence or qualifications. But if such an attitude disturbs you, look elsewhere.

If your potential physician is a member of a large group practice or HMO, there may be a patient representative or patient-relations department or similar office that will supply you some biographical information. Another source of information is the *Directory of Medical Specialists*(1). This lists physicians of all specialties by geographic location, alphabetically and by specialty. Although awkward to use because of its abbreviated codes, it does provide a minibiographic sketch and details of a physician's education, training, faculty status, and hospital affiliations. This volume is available in medical, hospital, and most public libraries.

A physician's schooling and training may have a lasting effect on his practice of medicine. The student who attended outstanding undergraduate medical colleges is likely to be among the brighter and harder working individuals. If his postmedical school internship and training were at a good university hospital, this suggests that he was high in his medical school class.

Regardless of the kind of practice he has, you should look for an indication that he is board certified—that is, has met the requirements and passed the examinations that have been established by the specialty board (see end of chapter). Any physician can declare himself a specialist in any area; board certification is documentation that he is in fact knowledgeable in his field. You may come across the designation "board eligible." This signifies that the physician has had the requisite training, but has not taken the examination. Some of the boards require a period of practice before the candidate can take the examinations—these may be outstanding younger physicians and are generally considered bona-fide specialists. If a physician has been in practice for years and is not board certified, this may mean that he has failed the examinations or that, for some reason, he has just never taken them. This should raise some questions in your mind.

If the physician you are considering is a full-time member of a medical-school faculty, he can be expected to be quite knowledgeable in his field and also have some skill in teaching, research, and administration. You may come across the designation "clinical faculty." The significance of this varies from medical school to medical school, but generally refers to a physician in private practice who maintains some connection with a medical-school faculty—usually as a part-time teacher or preceptor. This association may be fairly intense or may be on paper only, but it does suggest that the doctor has some interest in teaching, learning, and the intellectual side of the profession.

Your physician's hospital affiliations may be quite important. If he has *no* hospital privileges, this is quite suspect. It is in hospital practice that a physician's work is visible to his peers and administrators, so that hospital privileges per se indicate at least acceptable abilities. Increasingly, hospitals are defining more and more precisely just what a staff physician may do, on the basis of his training and demonstrated abilities. The details of a physician's hospital privileges is not, at present, generally available to the public.

A doctor's affiliation with a hospital may be of various kinds. He may be on courtesy staff, which means that he can admit patients to that hospital but that he is not very active or involved at that institution. He may have consulting privileges, which suggests that he meets that hospital's standards as a consultant in his field, but has in other respects the same relationship to the hospital as courtesy staff. He may be on active staff (or attending physician, or staff physician), which indicates that he is active in the life of the hospital—he attends meetings and usually educational programs, has committee obligations, etc. This, of course, allows closer scrutiny by his peers and is, in general, desirable. If he is on the active staff of a very good hospital, that is reassuring. If he practices in a locality with outstanding hospitals but is on the staff of only hospitals with a poor reputation, that would be some cause for concern.

Some physicians do research, publish articles in medical journals, or write or contribute to medical textbooks. This, of course, indicates a keen interest in a particular field, the ability to write, and the desire to communicate with other physicians, all desirable qualities. However, the physician's bibliography, if any, is not usually available in the sources discussed above—you would have to ask him, if you wanted to know that he has published.

It is possible that the most brilliant medical researcher may be unfit to treat human beings and that the relatively unlettered solo practitioner may be an unknown Osler—but, in general, choose the best trained doctor you can. The ideal physician would have gone to an excellent college or university, then an American medical school of high reputation, then trained in his specialty at a university-affiliated residency; he would be board-certified in his specialty and be on the active staff at the best hospitals in town; he would show some continuing interest in his professional growth by being active in teaching, research, or special studies.

Reputation

A physician's reputation, good or bad, may not be justified, but it is clearly worth noting. Unfortunately, a bad reputation is probably more reliable than a good one. A physician's reputation among his peers may be quite different from that among his patients. So if possible, check both sources. If you know any doctors who are familiar with the doctor in question, ask about him. You can try asking the administrator of the hospitals which he uses, although you will probably not get much information from that source. Most local medical societies and state licensing boards have a patient-relations office, and you may try to find out if there have been complaints about or charges against your prospective physician. Expect to hear nothing bad said; if you do find a problem, take heed.

If you can, talk to some of the doctor's patients. But keep in mind that a physician's popularity with his patients often has little to do with his competence. Almost every week there is a story of a doctor caught in some unethical conduct or dereliction of duty, whose many patients testify that he is a wonderful healer and a great person. A single disgruntled patient may downgrade a good doctor all over town, while a patient "saved" from a dread illness—more through the strength of his own constitution than the ministrations of his doctor—may sing praises unending. But if you hear the same report from multiple patients, good or bad, it is probably true.

Experience

There *is* no substitute for experience. Theoretically, the good physician should be able to recognize a condition he has never seen before, by virtue of his book knowledge and his deductive skills. And indeed, we all do recognize, from time to time, our first case of something. But recognizing disease is a little like recognizing a face. If you have never laid eyes on a person it may be difficult to recognize him even if you have read the most detailed account of his features, and even if you have seen photographs. But once you met that person face-to-face, you later recognize him instantly and positively. The physician who has seen and treated many cases of a disorder is definitely at an advantage. You should choose a doctor who has experience with your particular problem. His qualifications and training may make it plain, for example, that he is experienced in dealing with diabetes or heart disease. If you don't know how much experience he has, ask. You may have an unusual problem such as, say, industrial exposure to an uncommon chemical. If, as would be expected, your physician does not have experience with this problem, he should indicate a willingness to find out about it. Research and consultation can sometimes compensate for lack of experience.

Age, incidentally, is not necessarily a good indicator of experience. An older physician may have been making the same mistake for years, and call that experience. A young physician who has just completed four to seven years of intense hospital training may, on the other hand, have acquired a great experience in a short time.

In the case of the surgeon the issue of experience is quite critical, since the surgeon cannot ordinarily get help in the operating room if he suddenly finds the procedure beyond his experience. Indeed, in the case of surgery it has been well documented that surgeons who perform a given operation frequently have better results than do those who perform the procedure occasionally. This has been so well shown, in fact, that surgical societies have published some specific guidelines concerning the number of procedures that a surgeon needs to do to maintain adequate competence. The American College of Surgeons, for example, recommends that open-heart surgery teams should perform at least 150 operations a year. A team that performs fewer than that can be expected to have inferior results: more deaths, more complications, and longer hospital stays. It has been suggested that low-volume open-heart surgery units should, therefore, be closed. If you are scheduled for such surgery, find out how many such procedures are performed in that hospital. If the number is low, think twice about the surgeon and hospital.

The more specialized the surgical procedure, the more important this issue becomes. The most well-trained neurosurgeon, for example, cannot be expected to have superior results if, in the course of his first four or five years in practice, he has operated on only three or four cases of, say, the small, rupture-prone bulges (known as berry aneurisms) of the brain's small arteries. If you are faced with the need for this kind of critical surgery, you must find out the surgeon's experience, even if this is difficult or unpleasant. You may have to lean hard on the surgeon or the physician who is referring you to him—but you should find out.

Availability

Consider now your potential doctor's availability. He's not much good to you if you can't get to see him when you have to. Unless you have heard from other patients, it is hard to tell ahead of time how much or little trouble you may have in getting to talk to or see the doctor, or how long you can expect to wait in his (so aptly named) waiting room.

But you should be able to find out what kind of arrangements there are for nights and weekends. You don't want to call the office only to be connected with an answering machine that tells you to call an answering service, whose operators put you in touch, after a long wait, with the wrong doctor. But the solo practitioner always on call is rapidly disappearing or is gone; expect your doctor to have some kind of "coverage." If he is a member of a small group, that is probably ideal. There is a good chance that your own doctor will be on call, and even if he is not, each member of the group is familiar with the practices of the others, may even be familiar with your case, and clearly has a strong vested interest in providing you with good service. All these advantages become somewhat diluted by larger groups, since each doctor is on call less often, and you are likely to deal with a physician who is a stranger to you. Solo practitioners and small group practices may take turns taking each other's calls so that they can have some time off. This kind of coverage can work well but at times is somewhat casual, and communications between the doctors may not be ideal. Least desirable is the situation in which the doctor simply does not make any specific arrangements for off-hours calls and expects you to go to his hospital emergency room in case anything urgent comes up.

Ideally your doctor should practice not too far from your home or work. If the distance is great or the traffic likely to be snarled or the parking impossible, even the most "available" physician may in fact be quite inaccessible (especially if the patient is your screaming infant). He should be available by phone at any reasonable hour and have clearcut coverage arrangements for off-hours, with some arrangements for hospital emergency-room care in case of dire emergency.

Availability is one area in which the full-time member of a medical-school faculty may fall short. He has responsibilities not only to you and his other patients, but also to students, residents, his research, and administrative duties. He may see patients only one or two days a week, and frequently is unreachable after hours, leaving patients to rely on the emergency room for urgent problems. The subspecialist may also be frequently unavailable. On the other hand, physicians who offer primary care should be expected to be on call when you need them—most of the time.

Fees also affect availability—if they are too high, the doctor becomes inaccessible. Do not hesitate to ask, in advance, what the doctor's fees are. Be specific. Ask about the charges for the services you need. Many physicians now categorize their services according to CPT (Current Procedural Terminology). They usually include separate categories for new and old patients. Surgeon's fees are for consultation at various levels (comprehensive or complete, brief, intermediate, etc.). Surgical fees are determined by the type of operation. Medical doctors (internists and family practitioners) usually have four or five categories, including minimal visit, brief, intermediate, extended, and comprehensive. If you want a complete checkup by an internist, expect the comprehensive new-patient office-visit charge. Expect, too, charges for various tests (blood counts, cholesterol, electrocardiogram, etc.) and possibly procedures such as proctoscopic examination. If you only want the doctor to check your ear or treat your allergy or bursitis, make this known at the outset, so that the doctor doesn't provide you with a more extensive service than you want. Some physicians, especially internists, will insist on doing a complete physical on the first or at most second visit. If this practice (even though it has much to recommend it) is not to your liking, you will have to seek your medical care elsewhere. But it is better to find out before the visit. If the office staff is unwilling or unable to tell you the fees, be cautious. If the fees seem too high, compare them with the fees of comparably trained physicians.

Personality and Practice Style

Having considered the specialty, education, training, qualifications, and availability of your potential physician, you are still faced with the peculiar fact that this in no way assures you that you will be satisfied with him. This is because satisfaction depends heavily on the relationship that develops between the two of you, and this in turn depends on your personality and style too, but more on that later.

The physician's personality and practice style determine, among other things, how well he communicates with you, how he relates to you, and the role that he expects you to play in the professional encounter.

Doctors *should* be good communicators; the word "doctor" derives from the Latin word for "teacher." But your doctor may use jargon and technical language that makes him incomprehensible. This is sometimes a pompous affectation designed to make you feel inferior or to hide ignorance. But more often it is simply habit and laziness—the doctor has been speaking this way all his professional life, and so have his colleagues, and he barely knows any other way to speak. Or he may say very little at all. If you don't care about this, fine. But if understanding what the doctor is thinking and doing, understanding your medical problem, is important, this can be a critical issue. Your doctor may be a positive genius, but you will be unsatisfied if you are not satisfied by the way he communicates. Sometimes a direct request for a comprehensible explanation will do the trick—perhaps he doesn't know that he is being unclear. If the problem can't be cleared up, however, you will sooner or later find yourself looking for another doctor.

Some doctors are condescending and treat patients as if they were idiots. Amazingly, some patients don't seem to mind. Some of the most arrogant physicians I know have a devoted patient following. Gynecologists have come in for some very heavy criticism from feminist writers and press for their condescending and sexist attitudes. My own limited and admittedly subjective and unscientific observations would suggest that this has had a telling effect, and most gynecologists now, especially the more recently trained, seem a lot more aware of and concerned with their relationship to the patients.

You may look on your doctor as sort of a supereducated plumber. He has technical skills and knowledge which you expect him to apply. You see him for a specific complaint or problem, and you expect him to do what you want him to: examine and treat the ear infection; check the blood pressure; operate on the varicose veins. Some physicians don't mind that; others take a very different view of the matter and want to be advisers and teachers; they expect you to put your whole life history and, indeed, your very life, in their hands. If you and the doctor differ greatly on these issues, you are not going to stay together very long.

You may take the attitude the doctor knows best: Just tell me what to do—tests, medications, diet, surgery. You may not want to ask a lot of questions or play a major role in making medical decisions. After all, making medical decisions is what the doctor is trained and paid for. On the other hand, you may expect to take a major role in the medical decision making, and expect to learn the pertinent medical facts.

You will not be happy unless the doctor you choose is comfortable with your attitudes on these questions. There are some who insist on giving orders; there are others who seek a partnership with their patients. If you pick the wrong kind, things may not go well.

Ethnic, educational, economic, and personal factors may also affect your satisfaction with your doctor. Most doctors are wealthy, white, conservative males. If you aren't a member of that group, and if your vocabulary, experiences, and values differ greatly, it may be difficult to establish a satisfactory working relationship. Physicians are supposed to learn to communicate with and understand people of all walks of life; few can actually do so. It is surprising that, in spite of intimate contact with the poor during their training years, physicians can come away with little sympathy or insight. The poor have traditionally supplied physicians-in-training the experience they need to be able to treat the wealthy later. During that training young doctors spend long hours and longer nights at the bedside of the impoverished and unfortunate, witnessing their small victories, their pain and health. And yet, amazingly, many seem to learn little compassion and less understanding from these encounters. The most highly trained and well-qualified physician may have the sensibility of a baboon. Unfortunately, you may have no way of knowing this before meeting him.

Some personal characteristics of your potential physician should be mentioned. In general I would recommend ignoring race, sex, age, and ethnic background in choosing your physician. The stereotypes usually don't apply: There are stone-hearted female and nurturing male physicians; there are cautious, conservative young doctors and impulsive old ones. True, you may encounter physicians who are intolerant of your life-style or sexual preference, or you may come across one whose professional training and humanity has not overcome his bigotry or narrow-mindedness, and in these cases you will want to make a change.

After you have chosen your doctor—when you have come to his office or he to your bedside—the doctor-patient relationship begins. And this is, finally, an encounter between two strangers, with all its inherent complexities and uncertainties. And this is precisely why the correct choosing of a doctor is such a difficult exercise. Consideration of the issues discussed in this chapter may, however, increase the likelihood that the choice will be a felicitous one.

RECOGNIZED MEDICAL BOARDS

Listed below are the officially recognized specialties with some (I hope) pertinent or interesting comments.

Twelve boards are recognized by the American Board of Medical Specialties (which represents all the specialty boards listed below), and the American Medical Association Council on Medical Education. To become a certified specialist, a candidate must meet the requirements of the board, which usually consists of completing an approved training program and passing an examination.

American Board of Allergy & Immunology. Members of this board specialize in allergy testing and treatment. They are also experts in the many diseases that involve malfunction of the immune system, such as lupus and rheumatoid arthritis. These specialists deal with such common diseases as asthma, and rare ones such as agammaglobulinemia (the Bubble Boy). Some of these doctors are in the forefront of research on organ transplants. If you know that your problem is one of allergy, you may wish to consult an allergist.

American Board of Anesthesia. Anesthesiologists, of course, put you to sleep during your surgery. They also administer spinal anesthesia. Modern anesthetists, however, do far more. During difficult or prolonged surgical procedures, they monitor and establish control of virtually every vital function of the body. With their drugs and gases, with their catheters in multiple blood vessels and virtually every bodily opening, they control the rate and depth of breathing, the oxygen concentration in the blood, the blood pressure, the heart rate, the blood count, and even the brain's electrical activity. In the postoperative period, they monitor recovery and treat any complications. They are experts in cardiopulmonary resuscitation and are active in many aspects of medical research. They are teachers and counselors. They are experts in the management of chronic pain. If you need an anesthesiologist, the choice ordinarily will be made by your surgeon or the hospital.

American Board of Colon and Rectal Surgery. This was formerly the American Board of Proctology. These specialists extend their training, after studying general surgery, to acquire the high technical skills necessary to perform surgery in this complex and vital part of human anatomy. Your choice of such a specialist will depend on the availability of a colon/rectal surgeon, the nature of your problem, and your primary-care clinician or general surgeon. Many colon operations and surgery for hemorrhoids are commonly and competently performed by general surgeons.

American Board of Dermatology. Although many common skin disorders can be treated by primary-care specialists, refractory cases of common ailments (such as acne), or recognition and treatment of uncommon skin disorders require the somewhat arcane knowledge and nostrums of the expert. Dermatology is going through some great changes as new scientific research methods gradually supplant the traditional descriptive and empiric medicine. Skin disorders are sometimes a clue to inner bodily dysfunction, so the dermatologist has to be a competent all-around physician. This is another specialist whom you may wish to seek out for yourself.

American Board of Emergency Medicine. One of the newest specialities, this discipline arose for a variety of reasons: including modern advances in cardioplumonary resuscitation and other high-technological emergency treatments; fear of malpractice suits; the need for on-the-spot twenty-four-hour coverage; and the formation of independent physician groups which provide services to the hospital by contract. You will probably never seek out such a specialist, but there is a good chance you will sooner or later be treated by one, since these are the doctors who staff many hospitals' emergency rooms.

American Board of Family Practice. The modern transformation of the old GP, these physicians are highly trained in family medicine. However, they do only minor surgery, and most do not deliver babies. Their forte is primary care and care for the whole person, initial diagnostic evaluation, preventive medicine, and concern for the psychological and personal factors in health and disease. They are experts on the subject of what constitutes an appropriate checkup at various ages and often have vast experience in the treatment of diabetes, hypertension, and other chronic diseases. You may choose a family practitioner for your doctor, especially if you want one doctor for the whole family and all your needs.

American Board of Internal Medicine. The internist is the ultimate diagnostician, the intellectual of the profession, the clinician called upon in the complicated or obscure case. He embodies the scientific spirit in medicine, applying his knowledge of human physiology and the natural history of disease to the diagnosis and treatment of the sick patient. Medical knowledge has increased so rapidly in the last twenty-five years that this specialty has divided into many subspecialities. The internist who does not subspecialize is known as a general internist. His role has gradually changed from consultant to primary-care clinician. He is noted for his thoroughness and ability to detect the clues that indicate disease in its earliest form.

The practice of all internists rests on an intense two- or three-year residency program on the wards, or in the intensive-care units, emergency rooms, and clinics. The general internist continues to develop these skills, while the subspecialist takes a residency or fellowship in one of the subspecialties listed below.

CARDIOVASCULAR DISEASE. The cardiologist. Much more than the expert with the stethoscope, today's cardiologist regularly does heart catheterization, stress tests, coronary angiography, and even balloon angioplasty (dilating narrowed coronary arteries with an inflatable balloon). Some cardiologists will see you only if you are referred to them by other doctors, but some will be happy to see you without a referral if you have a cardiovascular problem.

CRITICAL CARE. The high-technology care of the modern intensive-care unit has become so complex that it has given rise to its own subspecialists. These are the men and women who deal with the desperately ill, whose survival depends on the monitoring and control of every life function and organ. Anesthesiologists, and some surgeons, may also be certified by this specialty board.

GASTROENTEROLOGY. The stomach specialist. These physicians specialize in the disease of the entire gastrointestinal system, which includes stomach, bowel, colon, liver, gallbladder, and pancreas. In addition to the diagnosis of difficult cases, these specialists can pass scopes into virtually any portion of the gastrointestinal tract for inspection, biopsy, or treatment. You might want to go directly to a gastroenterologist, but since many different conditions can cause abdominal pain or gastrointestinal symptoms, it is usually wiser to see a primary-care specialist and be referred to a gastroenterologist if necessary.

PULMONARY DISEASE. These physicians diagnose and treat diseases of the lungs including asthma, pneumonia, lung tumors, emphysema, bronchitis, and blood clots in the lung. Diagnostic tests include X rays, breathing tests, bronchoscopy (which allows the physician to look directly into the windpipe and bronchial tubes), and needle biopsy of various structures within the chest. You would not ordinarily see a pulmonary-disease specialist unless you have a severe or unusual pulmonary problem, or needed one of the special pulmonary tests.

ENDOCRINOLOGY AND METABOLISM. The specialty that deals with the endocrine glands such as the pituitary, thyroid, adrenal, ovary, testicles, and others. The endocrinologist's knowledge of the complex interactions of these glands, with their positive and negative feedback loops, allow him or her to define in ever greater detail how these glands control such crucial attributes as bodily size, sex differentiation, and even some aspects of personality. These physicians also specialize in the metabolism and the chemistry of the body, including such conditions as diabetes, gout, abnormalities of blood fats, kidney stones, and others. The initial diagnosis of an endocrine or metabolic disease will usually be made by your primary-care specialist who will refer you if necessary. If you know that you have an endocrine problem such as thyroid disease, or diabetes, you may wish to seek out your own endocrinologist.

HEMATOLOGY. The specialty dealing with disorders of the blood, including anemia, sickle-cell disease, bleeding disorder, and leukemia. These physicians are expert at obtaining and examining samples of bone marrow to assist in the diagnosis and treatment of these disorders. They often also specialize in cancer (see *Medical oncology* below).

INFECTIOUS DISEASE. Infectious disease involves every branch of medicine; all physicians treat some varieties of infectious disease. Infectious-disease specialists are usually called in on a case that is obscure, extremely complicated, or very difficult to treat. These men are the experts with the new and ever more numerous antibiotics; they know the nature and behavior of the common and uncommon infectious disease agents such as bacteria, viruses, spirochetes, and fungi. They commonly are involved in the care of patients with meningitis, infections on the heart valves, and complicated postoperative infections. You don't usually need an infectious-disease specialist to treat such common infections as a sore throat, pneumonia, or kidney infection.

MEDICAL ONCOLOGY. From the Greek *onko*, meaning "barb" or "hook," this specialty deals with the medical (not surgical) diagnosis and treatment of cancer. These specialists are expert in diagnosing cancer and treating patients with cancer chemotherapy. Because chemotherapy so often affects the blood and bone marrow, the specialties of medical oncology and hematology are often combined. The severe toxicity of some of the drugs, which may cause destruction of bone marrow, loss of hair, agonizing nausea and vomiting, and susceptibility to infection, is well known. Perhaps less well known is the increasing number of cancers that can be controlled and often cured by the expert use of some of these agents. Many of these agents are so new or so toxic that they are used almost exclusively by medical oncologists.

NEPHROLOGY. This subspecialty deals with disease of the kidneys. Kidney disease ultimately affects every organ system, so the nephrologist has to be a kind of superinternist to deal with myriad complications. These are the professionals who developed the artificial kidney, which has saved many from the prolonged torture of uremic death. The use of artificial kidneys is so complex that in most communities only nephrologists use them.

RHEUMATOLOGY. Not just rheumatism. Finding the cause of joint pain or swelling can tax any clinician's skills. There are literally dozens of causes of arthritis—from infection, to trauma, to hormonal problems, to disorders of the antibody system such that the body attacks its own joints. These cases often affect the arteries and thus every part of the body and every organ, including brain and kidney. For such cases and for the ordinary forms of arthritis that are extraordinarily unresponsive to conventional treatments, you may need a rheumatologist.

American Board of Neurologic Surgery. The neurosurgeon. Brain tumors, cerebral aneurism, head injuries, spinal-cord compression, some cases of slipped disk—these difficult cases require surgery that is treacherous and tedious, sometimes taking many hours, sometime requiring a microscope to minimize tissue damage. Neurologic tissue cannot regenerate, does not heal well, and is very sensitive to lack of glucose, blood, or oxygen. The neurosurgeon is forever "on the edge" with no margin for error. You will ordinarily not see a neurosurgeon until your condition is diagnosed by a primary-care physician or a neurologist who refers you.

American Board of Nuclear Medicine. Another specialist you are not likely to seek out on your own, this person deals with the radioactive materials of medical practice. These fall into two categories—diagnostic agents, which involve the administration of minute quantities of radioactive materials to measure function (as in a thyroid uptake), to obtain an image (as in a brain scan), or to measure blood flow (as in a lung scan), and the therapeutic agents, which involve the administration of much larger doses of radiation in order to destroy specific tissue. Examples are therapeutic doses of radioactive iodine to destroy cancerous or overactive thyroid tissue or the insertion into the uterus of radioactive rods to destroy cancerous tissue.

American Board of Obstetrics and Gynecology. Everyone is familiar with this specialty. In many communities only obstetricians now deliver babies. While office gynecology, including routine checkups, PAP smears, and contraceptive advice, is often provided by family practitioners, internists, and general surgeons, Band-Aid tubal ligation and many gynecological surgical procedures are done only by gynecologists. However, this specialty in its modern version encompasses much more and includes the following subspecialties:

GYNECOLOGIC ONCOLOGY. This specialty deals with the surgical treatment of gynecologic cancers, including cancer of the cervix, uterus, and ovaries.

MATERNAL AND FETAL MEDICINE. This specialty deals with all the ailments associated with pregnancy, as well as ailments of the fetus. It is now possible to recognize and sometimes treat abnormalities of the unborn baby. These abnormalities include hormonal imbalances, diabetes, abnormalities of the body's chemistry, and congenital deformities.

REPRODUCTIVE ENDOCRINOLOGY. Infertility can now be sometimes cured or overcome, using newer hormonal treatments, insemination techniques, and in-vitro fertilization (test-tube babies). Reproductive endocrinologists specialize in these treatments.

American Board of Ophthalmology. The eye doctor. Unlike the optometrist who prescribes eyeglasses, the ophthalmologist is a physician. He specializes in diseases of and surgery of the eye. The new high technology is very much present in this rapidly developing specialty. Laser beams, ultrasound, CAT scans, and microsurgery are all used in the diagnosis and treatment of eye diseases. Some aspects of ophthalmology are so difficult that they have given rise to informal subspecialties. Some ophthalmologists treat only the retina; some specialize in neuro-ophthalmology, which deals with the neurologic control of the eye movements and pupillary reflexes, and the formation by the brain of a single three-dimensional image derived from the impulses from each eye.

American Board of Orthopedic Surgery. Broken bones, tendon and muscle injuries, correction of scoliosis, surgical treatment of slipped disks, hand surgery. An orthopedist is a *very* good man to have around if you've been, say, in a motorcycle accident. Newer areas of orthopedic surgery include a very sophisticated brand of sports medicine, including arthroscopic joint surgery, which allows recovery in days instead of weeks or months. And now there are artificial hip and knee and finger joints to replace those destroyed by disease or injury.

American Board of Otolaryngology. You don't need an ear, nose, and throat specialist every day. But if you need ear surgery, or have a problem with your vocal cords, or have certain forms of mouth or throat cancer, seek out this person. More recently, otolaryngologists have been performing surgery to alleviate certain forms of the sleep-apnea syndrome, manifested by difficulty with breathing in sleep, and severe daytime drowsiness.

American Board of Pathology. The pathologist is another one of the doctors whom you may never see but who may affect you greatly. He examines the tissue removed during surgery and pronounces it benign or malignant, localized or invasive. And on his say-so the breast biopsy becomes a mastectomy or the planned removal of a lobe of the lung is found unnecessary. The pathologist is the director and overseer of the clinical laboratory in which all the blood and urine and spinal fluid and sputum samples are examined, analyzed, and measured. All manner of diagnoses depend on the pathologists' report, including ultimately the postmortem diagnosis.

American Board of Pediatrics. Everyone knows what a pediatrician is and does. As a parent you may choose a pediatrician for your child, or use a family practitioner; either one, if competent, can take care of your child. A family practitioner will be your first choice if you want one doctor to meet all or most of your family's needs. If, on the other hand, you are selecting a physician specifically for your child, you may be more inclined to select a pediatrician. If you do prefer a family practitioner, or if a pediatrician is not readily accessible, you may rest assured that if the situation required the special skills of a pediatrician, a competent family practitioner will make an early and appropriate referral.

Pediatrics has subspecialized much as internal medicine has, with neonatologists, pediatric rheumatologists, neurologists, surgeons, ophthalmologists, and many other subspecialties. Under most circumstances, if you need a pediatric subspecialist, your pediatrician will refer you.

American Board of Physical Medicine and Rehabilitation. These are the doctors to see if you have a problem with the mechanics of posture or movement. Some have become experts in sports medicine. They diagnose and treat scoliosis, muscle spasm, tendonitis, muscle injury, and the pains of biomechanical/dysfunction. The medicine/rehabilitation specialist is also expert at improving your function if you have an otherwise uncorrectable disability. They can fit (or, if necessary, design) a prosthesis so that gait, grip, or the ability to use an appliance, tool, or vehicle is restored.

American Board of Plastic Surgery. Facial surgery, cosmetic surgery (including breast reduction or augmentation), and, more recently, liposuction are some of the areas of their expertise. These surgeons help restore the damaged appearance and self-image of patients after injuries or cancer surgery, and correct congenital deformities.

American Board of Preventive Medicine. You will not usually choose a practitioner of this specialty. These doctors usually work in departments or public health or medical-school faculties. Their areas of concern include aerospace medicine, occupational medicine, and public health and epidemiology.

American Board of Psychiatry and Neurology. This board encompasses two very different fields: psychiatry and neurology. Neurologist- and psychiatrist-to-be both go to medical school for four years. After that their paths diverge, the psychiatrist taking a psychiatry residency and the neurologist a neurology residency. For board certification, however, they have to pass the same examination—the psychiatrist must know the anatomy, physiology, and disease of the nervous system; the neurologist must know the diagnosis and treatment of psychiatric disorders.

The neurologist deals with disorders of the brain, spinal cord, and nerves. Brain tumors, multiple sclerosis, dementia (including Alzheimer's disease), Parkinsonism, epilepsy, meningitis, and pinched nerves are some of the problems often referred to a neurologist. The neurologist can read brain wave recordings (EEG), do nerve tests of various kinds (evoked potentials, EMG), and other specialized diagnostic tests. Unless you have a previously diagnosed neurologic disease, you would probably not seek a neurologist without referral from a primary-care or other clinician.

The psychiatrist, of course, specializes in mental and emotional disorders. You may choose to select a psychiatrist yourself without referral. The psychiatrist is expert in psychotherapy and in drug treatment of mental and nervous disorders, and he can also hospitalize you, use electroconvulsive therapy when needed, and take care of many of the medical aspects of some disorders of mind and brain. Psychoanalysis, a very specialized and intense form of psychotherapy, is practiced by individuals who have trained in one of the few psychoanalytic institutes (a few nonphysician members are also trained in these institutes). Few psychiatrists are today so trained, for most psychotherapy practiced today is not psychoanalysis.

Many nonphysicians practice psychotherapy, making the choice of psychotherapist very difficult, but a detailed discussion of this subject is beyond the scope of this book. Among the practitioners are clinical psychologists, who have a Ph.D. in psychology plus a year of clinical training. Look for state licensure and certification by the American Board of Examiners in Professional Psychology or listing in the national Register of Health Service Providers in Psychology. Social workers with special training in psychiatric social work and therapy probably provide more psychotherapy than any other group. They have a master's degree or sometimes a doctorate in psychology or a related field. Expect accreditation by the Academy of Certified Social Workers. Psychiatric nurses can be expected to have a master's degree but have no formal certification or licensure for psychotherapy.

Additionally there are pastoral counselors, marriage counselors, sex therapists, and a variety of self-designated lay therapists. Some of these clinicians are very highly trained in psychotherapy and know also how to use various psychological tests to help diagnose mental disorders, while others have no training except for the therapy that they may have themselves received. The choice of clinician is not made easier by the intense rivalry that exists among some of these practitioners. Traditional psychotherapies include psychoanalysis, analytically oriented psychotherapy, Jungian analysis, and Adlerian analysis. Other therapies include EST, Gestalt therapy, bioenergetics, and Rolfing. Group therapies include psychodrama, traditional group therapy, family therapy, and transactional analysis. Additionally there are several cognitive-behavioral therapies including cognitive therapy, behavior modification therapy, and biofeedback.

American Board of Radiology. The old image of the radiologist looking at a series of static X rays is obsolete. Today equipment costing millions allows the radiologist to see into and through the body in amazing detail. Ordinary X rays are still used, of course, but these can be enhanced by computers that produce three-dimensional images that can be rotated, magnified, intensified, and otherwise manipulated. Even greater detail can be obtained by a non-X-ray technique called MRI (Magnetic Resonance Imaging). Detailed images of the brain, the interior of the eye, the abdominal cavity, or the spinal cord can be obtained painlessly. Further refinements of these techniques will soon allow the radiologist to "see" the metabolic activity of individual tissues, allowing an assessment of function as well as form. The sonogram is another non-X-ray image, especially useful because it is safe, painless, and inexpensive. It is the method especially useful in examining the fetus, the pelvic organs, and the gallbladder. The image is created by the variable reflection of ultrasonic sound waves. These and other new developments have made obsolete some previous painful or dangerous diagnostic techniques.

In addition to these diagnostic methods, radiologists are also therapists, using X rays, cobalt, and other radioactive energy sources to treat cancer and some other diseases. This is a specialty in its own right, and, indeed, radiology has developed numerous subspecialties including diagnostic, therapeutic, nuclear, and radiologic physics.

Any serious medical encounter that you have is likely to involve a radiologist. He or she will most likely be chosen by a hospital since most advanced radiologic methods require tons of equipment that exist only in hospitals or large clinics. There is a fair chance that you will never even see this specialist. In this circumstance you may need to rely on the assumption that a good hospital can be expected to have a good radiologist. Additional security about "your" radiologist comes from the fact that he is under the constant scrutiny of other doctors who depend on the accuracy of his reports.

American Board of Surgery. The physician to choose, of course, if you need your appendix or gallbladder removed, or a tumor. Also a good person to have if you are badly injured. He or she is perhaps the quintessential physician, the doctor in the heroic mode. Everyone knows what a surgeon does.

American Board of Thoracic Surgery. These physicians specialize in surgery of the chest, including the lungs, the esophagus, the great vessels, and the heart itself. They train for several years after completing a general surgery-training program. Modern understanding of human physiology, coupled with the great advances in anesthesiology, makes possible cardiac bypass surgery and heart transplants, which now have a predictable and reasonably high success rate. If you need a thoracic surgeon, you will probably be referred by another physician.

American Board of Urology. Another surgical specialty. Urologists are expert in surgery on the kidneys, the prostate gland, and the bladder. They also know how and when to insert a penile prosthesis for impotence, or perform a vasectomy. They are also the physicians to consult if you have a kidney stone that won't pass spontaneously. In the old days (before 1984) such a stone required surgery, but now, by using shock-wave lithotripsy, the stones frequently can be broken up into small harmless particles. In this procedure, the anesthetized patient is immersed in a tub, and underwater shock waves are focused on, and pulverize the stones.

You may have occasion to choose, or at least help choose, your urologist.

2

CHOOSING A HEALTH INSURANCE
Kurt Link, M.D.

In response to increasing pressure from all sides to control the cost of medical care, new kinds of medical insurance policies, and old kinds with new wrinkles, are rapidly appearing. The element that is new is the deliberate attempt to control medical practice. Health-insurance plans in the past did not attempt to influence medical decision making, but the new plans do, and some quite aggressively. The hope is that controlling medical costs will force medical decisions that make for a more efficient, rational, cost-effective, affordable, and hence accessible kind of practice. The fear is that patient's best interests will be subordinated to considerations of cost and profit. Many of the new plans restrict your access to specialists and other medical services, and greatly affect the style of medical practice.

The history of medical insurance in America is a search for the ideal plan—one which will pay the bill but not compromise the care.

HOW IT ALL GOT STARTED

Before 1932, formal health insurance was not readily available. Almost all medical service was fee-for-service. The patient paid the doctor (or the hospital) with his own money, and the quantity of services available depended on how much he needed and how much he could afford. As always, the poor received less care and the wealthy more. The physician's urge to provide many services was tempered by both the patient's reluctance to pay for services that he couldn't afford or that he thought he didn't need as well as the physician's fear of losing patients if his fees were too high. The inadequacies of this system became apparent during the Depression, when fee-for-service payments became an unreliable source of revenue. Furthermore, medicine was changing from a practice performed by independent professionals into a system dominated by institutions and specialized units that required large and stable revenues to operate. It became clear that there was a need to reduce the uncertain cash flow inherent in the irregularity of fee-for-service payments (1).

Some form of prepayment was required to free physicians, and more so hospitals, from the erratic behavior and fragile finances of patients. In 1929 a group of schoolteachers in Dallas, Texas, entered into an arrangement with Baylor Hospital whereby certain specified medical services would be provided in return for a prearranged monthly fee. The American Hospital Association adopted this experiment, and from it arose Blue Cross, the first modern health-insurance plan. This type of insurance with its conventional indemnity plan was welcomed by the medical establishment because it stabilized cash flow without interfering with medical practice or the setting of fees. The companies are merely fiscal intermediaries between patient subscribers, on the one hand, and hospitals and doctors on the other. They collect the premiums, which reflect the expenses and pay the bills. The insurance carrier has very little control of those expenses and even less on the quality of medical care.

But because this kind of health insurance puts no limit on the amount of medical services practitioners provide, costs tend to increase. This was particularly evident when the cost of medical care soared after the 1966 passage of Medicare and Medicaid. These insurances operated like Blue Cross and other indemnity plans—indeed they were often administered by those companies. By 1970 Washington became convinced that health-care costs were dangerously out of control.

This situation generated the Nixon administration's interest in prepaid, closed-panel group practices, euphemistically dubbed Health Maintenance Organizations. The name HMO was probably coined by Paul Ellwood, in Washington's Dupont Plaza Hotel, at a meeting on February 5, 1970. Paul Ellwood, who has been the greatest single champion of HMOs, was then director of the American Rehabilitation Foundation of the Sister Kenney Institute. He met with Nixon officials to formulate proposals for the control of runaway medical-care costs. Ellwood believed that, to this end, the administration should encourage prepaid care. He liked the words "health" because that suggested an emphasis on being well rather than sick, "maintenance" because of its connotations of preventive medicine and early diagnosis, and "organization" because of its neutral, benign tone.

While the hope was that such organizations would curtail medical costs, the crucial feature of these plans is that the provider has a strong incentive to minimize the cost of care. The HMO is paid a monthly capitation fee for each patient enrollee. The cost of providing all covered medical care is paid from these funds; the remaining monies are available for physician salaries or HMO profit.

Such plans have a long history. In 1929 the Ross-Loos Clinic was established in Los Angeles. The Ross-Loos plan organized a group of physicians to enter into a contract with the workers in the city's water department. For a prepaid fee, the physician group would provide care for the workers. In the same year the Elk City Cooperative was established in Elk City, Oklahoma. The Elk City Cooperative clinic went even further than Ross-Loos: This health-care plan was controlled by consumers, not physicians. This cooperative grew out of the desperate economic conditions prevailing in rural Oklahoma during the Depression.

These kinds of plans did not thrive at first, in part because of intense opposition from the medical establishment. Following World War II, however, the Kaiser-Permanante Medical Groups in California and the Health Insurance Plan of New York became major presences that kept an alternative to traditional health plans before the public. Since then, the HMO legislation of 1973 (the amendment to the Public Health Service Act known as PL 93-222 or Title XII-Health Maintenance Organizations) has stimulated a remarkable growth in the number of these plans. By 1980 there were well over 200 HMOs in America.

In recent years another variant of health insurance has appeared on the scene: the Preferred Provider Organization—PPO. This can be seen as a form intermediate between fee-for-service and the closed panel HMO. In a PPO, certain medical-care providers agree to accept a discounted fee; in return, the PPO encourages enrollees to use these (preferred) providers. Payment to the physician is still on a fee-for-service basis, albeit a negotiated one. The plan may contain financial incentives that encourage the physician to minimize cost of medical care. PPOs provide less control over costs and medical practice than do HMOs, but they allow greater patient choice and physician freedom.

Medicare for the elderly and Medicaid for the medically indigent are two multibillion dollar entitlement programs that were enacted in 1966. Both these programs are changing because of their unexpectedly great costs. Recent radical changes in the way Medicare reimburses hospitals has been associated with a dramatic decline in hospital utilization. The effect of this on the ultimate cost and outcome of medical care is so far unknown, but there can be little doubt that it is affecting the way physicians practice. In its early heyday, both Medicare and Medicaid were seen as a way, for the first time, to provide equal medical care for all American citizens. But in this time of budget deficits and spending cuts, that bright goal now shimmers like an unreachable, far-distant mirage.

The federal government also administers the Veterans Administration health-care system. Eligibility for VA care is determined by an imprecise and ever changing mix of medical and administrative criteria, subject to political influence and financial pressures. Top priority goes to veterans whose medical problems are attributable to their wartime military activities and require inpatient hospital care. Veterans who have civilian medical insurance have to decide when to use those benefits and when to use their VA benefits (if any). (If you think you might be eligible for care at the VA, you can contact one of the veterans advocacy groups or the eligibility officers who have offices in each VA hospital.) CHAMPUS is another, much smaller federal medical-insurance program for certain military personnel and retirees.

CONVENTIONAL HEALTH INSURANCE

There are two common forms of conventional health insurance: group health insurance and individual health insurance. Group health insurance, the more common type, is obtained through your employer (most commonly), or labor union or perhaps a professional, fraternal, religious, or alumni association. Usually, part or all of the cost of the premium is paid by the employer or organization. Important features of a group policy include the following: Your insurance coverage will lapse after you leave your job or organization unless you convert the policy to an individual one; you are automatically eligible for insurance as soon as you join the organization, although there may be some restrictions of coverage of preexisting conditions; your choice of plan is restricted to the one (or at most two or three) that the employer or organization offers.

Individual plans are those that you purchase through an agent or directly from the insurance company. There are now a great variety of plans from which you may pick and choose until you find one right for you. But before doing so you should review carefully the provisions regarding renewal and cancellation, looking for one that allows you to renew the policy at will. Many insurance companies may require you to have a physical examination and provide your past medical history and medical records to provide "evidence of insurability." Furthermore, there may be stringent restrictions on coverage of preexisting illness. In the case of a chronic disease, such as diabetes or high blood pressure, such restrictions may make the insurance all but worthless, since almost any ailment you may have might be attributed directly or indirectly to the preexisting condition.

Benefits and Costs

A typical conventional health insurance (group or individual) policy today covers the following expenses:

Basic Benefits

Hospital benefits—covers all costs incurred during a hospital stay, including room and board, laboratory and X-ray fees, medications, and treatments. If there is an extra charge for a private room, this may not be covered unless a private room is medically necessary.

Medical benefits—covers nonsurgical doctor's fees in and out of the hospital, and outpatient X-ray and laboratory fees. (These outpatient costs are sometimes covered by major medical policies—see below—and are not considered part of the basic benefits.)

Surgical benefits—covers surgical fees.

Major Medical Benefits

Provides coverage beyond the basic benefits. Each feature you select may increase your premium. These benefits may include the following:

Maternity benefits.

Care for catastrophic illness, especially for hospital expenses that go beyond the limits of the basic coverage.

Medications.

Medical equipment and appliances.

Nursing home care.

Private duty or other special nursing care.

Psychiatric care beyond that covered by basic benefits.

All these benefits have important restrictions. The number of hospital days allowed is usually limited. The limitation is such that if you have any ordinary illness, you will be fully covered, but if you suffer a medical disaster that requires months of hospitalization, your policy may be inadequate, and you may be financially destroyed. If coverage for catastrophic illness is one of your options, you should consider it. If it is not an option, you should consider buying an additional policy for catastrophic illness. Such policies are usually not very expensive because the company has to pay only after your basic benefits have been exhausted, and this is rare.

Surgical benefits are also limited. The insurance company has a maximum fee that it will pay for any surgical procedure. This is commonly referred to as a "usual and customary fee," or UCR (usual, customary, and reasonable) and is supposed to be based on the prevailing fees in your community. Each plan has its own version of these fees, and they may vary considerably. If your surgeon's fees are greater than the maximum fee your health insurance allows, you will have to pay the difference, unless you can get your surgeon to agree to accept the insurance payment as full-payment. Reaching such an agreement with your surgeon may be greatly complicated by a very peculiar practice common to the insurance companies: They do not divulge their fee schedule and will not tell you or the surgeon how much they will pay until after the surgery has been performed and the bill submitted. This supposedly discourages surgeons from always charging the maximum that the company will allow. It also makes it impossible to compare one plan's surgical benefits with another's.

Outpatient medical services are frequently limited. Checkups, periodic physicals, and all kinds of preventive medical care may not be covered. If these aspects of medical care are important to you, this may be a crucial limitation to your policy. Most policies will cover routine PAP smears once a year, but may exclude complete physicals, immunizations, mammography, screening proctoscopy, and screening laboratory tests. Your policy may only pay for tests that are required for the evaluation of a specific condition, for example, mammography will be paid for only if the doctor feels a lump, proctoscopy only if there are bowel symptoms or bleeding. This unfortunate feature of many insurance policies may encourage you (or your physician) to come up with a bogus diagnosis so that the services will be covered. This can lead to a situation that is uncomfortable for both of you and may interfere with your relationship.

A cost-sharing feature, if present, is another limitation to your coverage. Plans without cost-sharing provisions provide so-called first-dollar coverage; you pay nothing. Plans with cost-sharing provisions require you to pay some out-of-pocket expenses. There are three common forms of cost sharing:

Deductible. A deductible feature requires you to pay a fixed sum before your coverage starts. For example, you may have to pay the first $100 of medical bills; only after that will your insurance company pay. Usually you have to pay the deductible each year. The deductible may apply to the family as a whole or to individual members. There may be a separate deductible for various services. For example, there may be a medication deductible, a doctor's office fee deductible, and a hospital deductible.

Copayment. A copayment requires you to pay a fixed amount for each service provided. For example, you may have to pay $3.00 for each office visit. There may be copayments for a variety of other services as well. The list can be extensive.

Coinsurance. Coinsurance requires you to pay a proportion of the medical expenses. For example, your policy may pay for only 80 percent of the hospital bill. This kind of cost sharing can be the most costly. Furthermore, it is unpredictable. The amount you will have to pay out of pocket cannot be anticipated—it depends entirely on the total cost of medical services. A prolonged hospital stay could leave you with a very large bill indeed, even if your insurance pays 85 percent or 90 percent of the bill.

In most policies all three cost-sharing features come into effect together. Consider an ordinary, five-day hospital stay that costs (let's be modest) $2,000. If your plan has a $100 deductible, plus a $10 per day copayment, and a 20 percent coinsurance on the balance (these are common to many policies), you would be required to pay $520. Often the cost-sharing proportion changes as the bill gets higher, making it either more or less costly, depending on the circumstance. But unless the insurance pays 100 percent, a long hospitalization can mean a large coinsurance payment.

If you choose a policy with large cost-sharing features, the premium theoretically should be less than for a policy with small cost-sharing expenses. Estimating the total cost of your health care, therefore, depends on weighing the cost-sharing expenses against the presumably lower premium. Unfortunately, this is a gamble, since, as we have seen, many of the cost-sharing expenses are unpredictable. Of course, if your premium is being paid by your employer, that too must be taken into account.

The cost to society of conventional health insurance is not necessarily reflected by the premium. This kind of insurance encourages doctors to provide services whether needed or not and may encourage hospitalization by providing better coverage for in-hospital than outpatient care. As a physician, the more I do for you, the more I will make. You will not likely object to the provision of any needed covered services, since it is the insurance company that is paying the bill.

In order to collect your benefit payments, you will usually have to submit a claim form. You will have to fill out your part, and you will have to get your physician or his staff to fill out their part. If your physician accepts payment directly from the insurance company (and then bills you for the remainder), that makes life much easier for you. If he insists on billing you directly, you may have to put up the money and then wait for the insurance check.

Freedom of Choice and Style

So much for the benefits and cost. What about freedom of choice? Of the various kinds of health insurance, conventional health insurance restricts your choice of health care provider the least. It does not influence your medical care in any way. It does not even attempt to do that. The insurance company is not in the business of providing medical care at all. It acts as a fiscal intermediary; the company collects the premiums and pays the provider. Period. Hence, the term "third party payor." You can see any doctor or any kind of specialist you choose. You can pick and choose or change physicians at will. You can be hospitalized in any (appropriately licensed) hospital you wish. You will be covered equally well wherever you are in the country or even in the world. Your physician knows that any necessary care will be covered; he is free to treat or prescribe for you as his medical judgment dictates.

Conventional health insurance has little effect on the style of your medical care. If you like to see your personal physician in his private office, your insurance company will pay just as well as if you go to a large clinic or teaching hospital or other institution.

Thus, conventional health insurance provides medical coverage with well defined limits, has a relatively low premium, gives you almost complete freedom in choosing your doctor(s) and hospital(s) but may require significant out-of-pocket expenses.

HMO—HEALTH MAINTENANCE ORGANIZATION

HMOs are organizations that provide comprehensive health services to a defined population for a prepaid, capitated premium. When enrollment time comes at work and you are presented with brochures describing both a conventional health insurance plan and an HMO, the fundamental difference between the two systems may be obscured by relatively similar benefits and premiums. But the differences are there, and they are important.

Conventional health insurance, as we saw, does not provide or influence medical care and tends to reward providers for providing many services. The HMO, on the other than, is *the* provider of medical care and has a financial incentive to minimize health care costs. The HMO receives a fixed sum each month for every enrollee. This is the capitation fee. In return, the HMO provides all covered health services. If the cost of providing care is less than the total capitation income, there is a profit for the HMO. If the cost of providing care is more, there is a loss. The capitation fee is the same if the enrollee gets no medical care or is in an intensive care unit at $1,000/day. Thus the HMO has a financial interest in keeping costs low.

With these features in mind, let us now look at an HMO the way we looked at conventional health insurance—the benefits, the costs, the effects on freedom of choice and practice style. For ease of discussion I will assume that we are examining a federally qualified, staff model HMO, which is the purest form of HMO. The medical staff is housed in a central medical building; occasionally there are satellite offices in the surrounding community. The physician and the rest of the staff are salaried, full-time employees of the HMO. The physicians are not directly affected by the day-to-day cost of medical care, but in the long run, of course, their financial success depends on the success of the HMO. All their patients are HMO patients, and they see no others. We will later compare the staff model HMO to the other two common forms of HMOs—group models and IPAs—and discuss the significance of federal qualification.

Benefits and Costs

The benefits provided by HMOs generally exceed those provided by conventional health insurance.

    Basic benefits—the same as conventional health
        insurance.
    Major medical benefits—the same as conventional
        health insurance
    Maternity care
    Mental health services
        outpatient and (sometimes) limited inpatient care
        chemical dependency treatment
    Preventive services
        periodic physical examinations
        immunizations
        vision and hearing examinations for
            children
    Allergy testing and treatment
    Health education
        dietician services
        diabetic teaching
        cardiac teaching
        stress management
        smoking cessation clinics
    Additional optional benefits may include
        Prescription medication plan
        Prescription spectacles
        Dental care
        Medical appliances and equipment
        Home health care
        Skilled nursing facilities, extended care facilities, and long-term reha-
            bilitation services.

There are fewer limits to these benefits in an HMO than in conventional health insurance although the need for catastrophic insurance coverage may remain the same. Many months of hospitalization or a prolonged psychiatric hospitalization can outstrip your benefits. Maternity benefits are fully covered but may apply only to pregnancy that occurred after enrollment. Surgical fees

Choosing a Health Insurance

are fully covered. Indeed, you will never receive a bill from the surgeon or any other doctor you see in the HMO.

Outpatient medical services are all covered. These include immunizations, periodic health checkups, and all outpatient care: laboratory, X ray, physical therapy, all screening and health-maintenance care, including mammograms, PAP smears, EKGs, and any other tests that you need.

In an HMO there is virtually no paperwork for you. You do not have to fill out or mail any claim forms; you never have to wait for a check to arrive; you will never find a doctor's bill in your mailbox.

There is little or no cost sharing in an HMO. There is never a deductible or coinsurance. There may be a small copayment requirement such as $3.00 for an office visit. Such copayments are designed more to discourage unnecessary office visits than to raise revenue.

The cost of belonging to an HMO depends almost entirely on the premium. Because there is first dollar coverage (or close to it), you will have little or no expense beyond the premium. Furthermore, although the benefit package tends to be rather rich, the premiums may be quite competitive or only slightly higher than conventional health insurances'. But even high premiums have to be weighed against the opportunity for covered frequent office visits, PAP smears, mammography, health checkups, or large prescription bills.

Many health planners try to encourage the development of HMOs because they do, in fact, provide medical care at a lower cost. Many studies have shown this to be true. The reduction in costs is largely due to decreased hospital costs. This, in turn, is due to fewer hospital admissions and shorter stays (2). HMO physicians are under considerable pressure from their peers and utilization committees (3) to admit only those patients who cannot possibly be treated at home, and to get patients home as soon as possible.

Patients with conventional health insurance, one study found, have surgery five times more often than HMO patients (4). Some surgery may be unnecessary, but even if that is taken into account, HMO patients still have fewer operations. This would be expected if patients who choose HMOs are in good health to begin with, but does not seem to be the whole explanation (5). Other unknown factors appear to be at work.

HMO hospital costs may also be diminished if the HMO, because of its volume, can negotiate lower per diem hospital fees, or if it owns its own hospital.

Freedom of Choice and Style

HMOs restrict your freedom of choice of provider. You are required to use the HMO physicians, offices, and hospitals. As we discussed in an earlier chapter, choosing a physician is not easy. Everyone wants a qualified physician, and HMO physicians seem as well qualified as fee-for-service practitioners. But there are factors other than professional training which have to be taken into account. If you are a member of a relatively large HMO, there should be no great problem in choosing a primary-care physician to your liking because of the relatively large number to choose from. Even here there is potential for trouble, however, because you may not be free to change primary-care physicians without an explanation; more than one change may be resisted greatly. But problems in choosing a doctor are more likely to occur in the case of specialists, since even the largest HMO may have only one specialist in certain fields such as neurology or ear-nose-and-throat. In that case you may be required to deal with a physician you don't like.

Many HMOs will not pay for a specialist's service unless you have been referred by your primary-care doctor. The purpose of this is to make sure that referrals are appropriate and necessary, and coordinated with other aspects of your care. So if you are in the habit of deciding for yourself when, for example, to see a cardiologist or a urologist, this stipulation may cause trouble. But, on the plus side, the staff model HMO eliminates the financial barrier to referrals. And referrals are easy for your primary-care physician to make, either formally or over a cup of coffee or during a hallway conference.

You will have to use the HMO offices, which may not be convenient for you. If you are out of town, you may need to get authorization for any but emergency care before being attended to. Furthermore, the HMO may require you to return to your HMO service area at the earliest possible time. So if you do a lot of traveling, this may be a significant problem.

Your choice of hospital is also restricted. You must use the HMO-owned hospital if there is one, or else a hospital with which the HMO has a contract. This hospital may be selected more for its low rates than for its quality, and you may find that you are not using the hospital you would like.

The staff model HMO has a great impact on practice style. One of the advantages is that all your medical services are provided under one roof. Consultations are easily made, and the presence of a single medical record makes it possible for each clinician caring for you to be aware of your whole health picture. It is much easier to avoid the fragmentation of medical care so common in conventional medical settings.

You should be able to count on reaching a doctor at night or on weekends because a well-organized HMO has an on-call roster with appropriate backup call. Inherent in the virtues of such a system, however, is the great likelihood that you will reach a doctor you don't know just when you need your own doctor most. This brings up the issue of how the doctor-patient relationship is affected by an HMO. Theoretically, at least, the influence could be profound.

Consider that in the conventional system you pick out your doctor, you go to see him, and he then agrees to take on your case. Either party can withdraw at will at any time. (It may be necessary for you to have other medical care available before your doctor can withdraw from the case.)

The HMO scenario is different. First you choose your insurance plan. The choice of doctor comes second; often you will have been assigned to a total stranger. I have practiced in my own offices and as an HMO employee. It has always been my habit to ask new patients how they chose to see *me*. The usual answer is that they were referred by a patient or another doctor or an emergency-room staff or even the yellow pages. But when the answer is "because I have X insurance," I feel a twinge of discomfort. But as an HMO doctor I have no choice in the matter—you have paid your premium, you are entitled to care, and I cannot refuse. I may request you to transfer to another doctor if the relationship is intolerable, but I cannot do this very often. In an extreme case, if the HMO becomes convinced that you are abusing the system, it may be possible to disenroll you. But this almost never happens.

Another feature of the staff model HMO is the centralized medical building, which is often referred to as a clinic. The staff may be so large that its members do not even know each other; certainly they do not know you. As the facility gets larger, it tends to get more impersonal and institutional. Some clinics establish more or less autonomous modules to create a more intimate and personal environment, but often the feel of clinic persists.

Group Model and IPA

So far we have been discussing the staff model HMO. Another model is the group practice model. In this case, an established fee-for-service multi-speciality group practice agrees to provide medical services to HMO subscribers for a capitated fee. Such a group has already demonstrated its ability to attract fee-for-service patients. The HMO will require that its enrollees be treated no differently from the fee-for-service patients. But if the capitation is such that physicians are treating more fee-for-service patients, there is the possibility of developing a dual standard of care. On the other hand, a group model practitioner may be partly insulated from the financial pressure of the HMO, since the capitation is only a part of his income.

In addition to staff model HMOs and group practice models, there is the IPA (Independent Practice Association) model. An HMO owner—which can be an insurance company, a Blue Cross/Blue Shield organization, or a hospital—contracts with individual practitioners to provide services in their own offices. Usually, any qualified physician can be a participating doctor.

As a physician in an IPA-HMO, I am paid a capitation fee and so have the typical HMO financial incentives to control the cost of care, but some of the efficiencies and controls of the other HMO types are sacrificed. In return, however, you and I have the conveniences of using my smaller, private, neighborhood office, and there is less restriction of choice of physician and hospital. The covered benefits and other features are similar to those of the other kinds of HMOs.

Federally Qualified

If you are thinking of enrolling in an HMO, find out if it is federally qualified. To become federally qualified, an HMO must meet the requirements of the Health Maintenance Act of 1973 (PL 93-222). The HMO must

>   Provide a rich benefit package.
>   Base its premium on a broad representation of the community.
>   Have strong HMO member representation on its governing board.
>   Have a utilization review and quality assurance program.
>   Have grievance procedures for enrollees.
>   Guarantee that reenrollment or expulsion from the HMO will not be based on the member's health or need for medical services.
>   Provide continuing medical education for the health professionals.
>   Not have more than 75 percent of its enrollees from a medically underserved population (thus demonstrating its ability to attract fee-for-service patients).
>   Provide services twenty-four hours/day seven days/week.
>   There must be at least thirty days in each year during which you are allowed to enroll.

Such certification requires periodic inspection by federal officials, and considerable administrative effort and paper work (6). Many HMOs nonetheless choose to become federally qualified because they are then eligible for federal grants and loans, which can be crucial during the early years of operation. More importantly, federal qualification increases HMO access to subscribers because of the "dual choice option," which requires any organization with at least twenty-five employees to offer an HMO plan as an alternative to any traditional health plan, if at least twenty-five of its employees reside in the HMO's service area.

If your HMO is federally qualified, you know it will have the benefits and features noted above. If it is not federally qualified, it may be as good or better, but then again it may not. So you had better look closely at the benefits and services it offers.

Quality of Care in Conventional vs. HMO Systems

So far we have been comparing conventional health insurance with HMOs in regard to costs, benefits, freedom of choice, and practice style, but have said nothing about the quality of care. Let me begin this discussion by concluding: There is no *consistent demonstrable* difference in the quality of care between the two systems. There is abundant literature on this subject; a single computer search provided me with 151 citations. Some of this literature makes fascinating reading. Some of it is polemical if not hysterical. HMO advocates, usually of relatively left political inclination (but note the Nixon administration's position), say it is time to put a stop to a medical system that benefits the rich and further impoverishes the poor, that present-day medical care serves the medical establishment, not patients, that physicians profit from the misery and misfortune of their patients. They say that the HMO can bring a rational, efficient, and safe medical practice to all citizens, that HMO physicians have a vested interest in the health of their patients instead of their sickness.

HMO opponents, usually of right-wing persuasion and/or members of the medical establishment, say that HMOs seek to control the practice of medicine, destroy the patient-doctor relationship, and put cost considerations before consideration of quality of care. They say HMOs will be the destruction of the practice of medicine and the health of the nation.

A look at the data leads to much more modest conclusions. Part of the problem is figuring out how, in fact, to measure (or even define) quality of care. In an earlier chapter we saw that it is difficult to measure the performance of one physician; it is much more difficult to measure the performance of a whole system of medical care.

Quality of care is commonly evaluated by looking at three aspects of medical practice: (1) outcome, (2) structure and (3) process. The *outcome* of medical care is intuitively the most direct and clear-cut way of evaluating quality of care. But how is one to measure outcome? Death rates and longevity are the obvious, easily measured, unequivocal end points. The trouble is, as has been noted, much of medical care does not affect death rates or life expectancy. Many patients get better by themselves, and many patients die no matter how good the care. So even if there is a difference between the two systems of care, that difference may be undetectable.

Another measure of outcome is the number of days spent in hospital. But questions of interpretation immediately arise. Do more hospital days mean more sickness and poorer quality of care, or does it mean more and better care? The question is unanswered, and so this "measure" is not much good, either. Other outcome measures include missed days of work, complications and recurrences of diseases, and functional disability. The usefulness of these and many other outcome measures are diminished because it is so difficult to compare two medical-care systems. For one thing, the patients in the two systems are unlikely to be the same (7). Suppose HMOs attract healthier patients? Of course their "outcome" is going to be better (8). If one system eliminates financial barriers to medical care, outcomes may be affected—but does this apply to individuals who can afford fee-for-service care? Suppose one system is better for younger patients while another is better for older patients. When overall results are examined, such differences may be "averaged out" and so become undetectable.

Even if all these obstacles can be overcome, a difference in outcomes of, say, a few percentage points may take years to become measurable and might take decades to become statistically significant.

Another way to measure quality of care is to look at the *structure* of medical care. This method assumes that quality of care is directly related to the quality of the staff and facilities. For example, if all the clinicians have been trained at premiere institutions, and if the patient-clinician ratio is low, and if the facilities are modern, then the quality of care is judged to be good. Although HMO physicians are younger and are willing to be salaried employees rather than solitary entrepreneurs and may have other distinguishing personality traits (9), no obvious difference in overall qualifications has been demonstrated. But neither has there been good data (10). And even if there were good data, the measurement would be derivative—we would still not know for sure if the quality of care is better.

The third common way of assessing quality of care is to look at the "process" of care. This method assumes that quality can be assessed by examining the manner and quantity of services provided. For example, what percentage of patients have had a complete physical? How often are a rectal exam or PAP smear included in the exam? Are immunizations fully utilized? How long does it take to get an appointment for a routine visit and for an emergency?

Analyzing the process of care brings up at least two problems. The available data comparing the two health-care systems is sketchy, and there is no certain connection between process and outcome, which is still what we really want to know about. This is demonstrated by a 1978 (11) study comparing how urinary tract infections are handled by a prepaid group practice or individual practitioners. The researchers found that the process of care was better in the prepaid group practice; certain tests, especially cultures of the urine, were more appropriately utilized. But the study was designed only to examine process. The authors conclude that "no convincing evidence exists that patient outcomes are improved by . . . use of . . . urine cultures."

Keeping this framework of outcome, structure, and process in mind, let us review a few of the studies comparing the quality of care in fee-for-service or conventional health insurance with that of HMOs. An early study (8) compared the HMO to an "ideal standard" and not to conventional health insurance. The researchers found serious deficiencies in diagnosis and therapeutic outcomes for the following conditions: contraception, depression, hypertension. But they also noted that difficulties in data collection and deficiencies in the basic methodology made their findings of questionable significance.

A 1982 study of patterns of surgical care (12) showed the usual lower rate of surgery for HMO patients but identical "biological outcomes." Similarly, a very good study (13) comparing HMO and fee-for-service obstetric practice found that for "virtually every outcome measure (both for child and mother) there was no difference between the health maintenance organization and fee-for-service groups." There were more Caesarean section births among the fee-for-service patients, but the reason for this was unknown, and it did not seem to have any effect on overall quality of care.

The results of the most recent, and by far the best comparison of fee-for-service to HMO care, were published in 1987 (14). Thanks to funding from the RAND corporation, it was possible to perform a true experiment that avoided many of the usual obstacles to a good study. Approximately 1,500 patients were randomly assigned to either an HMO or fee-for-service group. Certain indicators of health were measured at the beginning of the study and again at the end, three to five years later. Twenty different "health status measures" were examined. These included such things as breathing capacity, EKGs, vision, and blood sugar. This study showed once again that HMO patients have less surgery and fewer hospital days, but this made no demonstrable difference in outcomes of medical care. HMO patients tended to be somewhat less satisfied because services were perceived as less personal. The authors finally "conclude that there were no major differences in measures of chronic illness or its effect on pain or worry in health practices between" the HMO and fee-for-service systems.

So I return to my conclusion: There is no consistent demonstrable difference in quality of care between fee-for-service and HMO care. Of course not all HMOs are equal, just as not all practitioners are equal, and the specific choices available to you may suggest that your care *would* be better in one or the other system. But, in general, if you are trying to decide whether or not to enroll in an HMO, the decision will have to be based on factors other than quality of care.

PPO—PREFERRED PROVIDER ORGANIZATIONS

HMOs are one kind of "managed" care. PPOs are another. Both these systems seek to influence or manage the whole process of medical care through administrative control and financial incentives. The goal is to provide care of such cost and quality that it will compete successfully in the health-care marketplace. PPOs are often described as intermediate between HMOs and fee-for-service care. As a PPO enrollee you can expect to have some, but not all, of the benefits of an HMO, but you can also expect to experience some, but not all, of the disadvantages of an HMO. (If you are *very* interested in this subject, you can read the recent Peter Boland guide to PPOs, 1,117 pages [15].) In the PPO system, the insurance contracts with individual practitioners (or a group or a hospital), who agree to provide medical care for enrollees at a predetermined and usually discounted rate. The practitioners agree to abide by the PPO rules, which may include controls over the ordering of tests, admission to the hospital, and referral to specialists. In return, the practitioner is designated a preferred provider, which carries the promise of more patients.

The benefits provided by PPOs vary considerably, but resemble those for conventional health insurance, sometimes with additional features such as well-baby care and certain preventive or screening measures (i.e., PAP smear, mammography).

The cost of care in a PPO that is functioning well will be less than in the fee-for-service model, but probably not as low as in a staff-model HMO. The cost to you as a patient may be hard to determine. The premium will often be quite competitive with other insurances, but a cost-sharing arrangement, as in conventional health insurance, is common. Your actual cost of medical care, therefore, will depend in part on how many services you require. As we have noted before, this is often unpredictable. You will have additional costs if you choose to use a provider who is not a preferred provider (see below). In theory, at least, the cost of care will be less than for a comparable conventional health-insurance program.

Your choice of physician is restricted in a PPO. You will be encouraged to choose a preferred provider—one who has, as we have noted, agreed to provide care at a predetermined, usually discounted rate. If you choose a physician who is not a preferred provider, it will cost you money. If there is no copayment for a preferred provider, there may be one for a nonpreferred provider. If there *is* a copayment for a preferred provider, there may be a coinsurance of, say, 10—20 percent for a nonpreferred provider. Selecting a preferred provider may not be a great problem when it comes to choosing your primary-care physician, because, unlike the closed-panel staff-model HMO, many—indeed almost any—physicians may sign up with the PPO. There is thus a fair chance that your regular doctor will be a participant.

The same issues apply to your choice of subspecialist. You may have a strong financial incentive to select a participating subspecialist. As in the HMO system, the choice in this case may be quite narrow, especially in the rarer subspecialties where choices are inherently limited anyway. Furthermore, your insurance may not pay at all unless you are referred by your primary-care physician. Some PPOs penalize the primary-care physician for making referrals, so problems may arise. One common arrangement is for the insurance company to establish a fund, called a referral pool, for each primary-care physician. The cost of any referral is paid from this fund. At year's end, any money left in the pool is distributed, in part, to the primary-care physician. As a primary-care physician I am, in this way, discouraged from making referrals. I hope, and believe, that this will encourage me to avoid unnecessary referrals, but will not interfere with the best interests of you, my patient. But the potential for mischief is there.

If you are considering enrolling in a PPO, I suggest that you try to find out if your primary-care physician will be at financial risk (and how much risk) if he makes referrals. Such a sophisticated inquiry will not make you popular with the insurance representative—who, indeed, may not even know the answer. But if you don't mind being considered a troublemaker, you may find out some useful information.

Your choice of hospital will be restricted, since the PPO will usually have an arrangement with one or several hospitals at which it gets favored treatment. The issues here are the same as in the case of hospital choice in the HMO, except that the PPO may have a larger number of affiliated hospitals.

One of the advantages of the PPO over the HMO pertains to practice style. This, of course, is a highly individual matter. If you prefer a personal relationship with a doctor who likes to run his own practice in his own office, then the PPO arrangement may be a good compromise between fee-for-service care and an HMO. As we have noted, the PPO physician does practice in his usual style, except that he is encouraged to do so as economically as possible. On the other hand, you may view your physician as a highly trained technician whom you hire to fix whatever you have determined needs fixing. You may feel that you have lived with and in your body for decades, that you are the real expert here, that you don't need your doctor to be a counselor or father-figure or friend. A relatively impersonal arrangement that provides you with an extensive menu of medical services may be what you consider ideal. A large HMO may, in that case, be exactly your cup of tea.

PPOs are relatively new in the health-care market. Some observers believe that they are a way station to HMOs; others believe that they are the wave of the future. Their history is too short to draw any conclusion (16). For now, it might be a good idea to find out how long your particular PPO has been in existence for some have already failed (just as HMOs, conventional health insurances and other business ventures sometimes fail).

MEDICARE

Medicare is a health-insurance program administered by the U.S. Government for people sixty-five and older, and for some disabled persons under age sixty-five. The benefits are paid for by Social Security taxes. In its beginning in 1966, Medicare payments to physicians were based on usual and customary fees, and payments to the hospitals were based on the cost-plus charges whereby hospitals were paid their cost plus a variable percentage thereof for their profit. Thus, virtually all citizens sixty-five or older had access to first-class medical care. In the ensuing two decades, however, there has been a decrease in the benefits, and an increase in the cost to patients, and restriction of payments to physicians and hospitals. These changes have been made necessary by the unexpectedly high cost of the program and the increasing resistance of the public to further increases in Social Security taxes. So hospital management now tries to get Medicare patients discharged at the earliest moment, and physicians are paid less for caring for Medicare patients than for fee-for-service patients. In spite of these limitations, this program is the remaining jewel of the social legislation passed during the Great Society days of the 1960s.

The Medicare legislation established two different insurance programs: Part A for inpatient hospital costs and Part B for outpatient medical costs. These really are two separate programs, and so I will discuss them separately.

Part A covers hospital expenses. Almost everyone over age sixty-five is eligible. If you do not have sufficient work credits to be eligible, you may purchase Part A hospital insurance by signing up for it at your local Social Security office during the three months before you are sixty-five or during the first three months of any year thereafter. You may then also buy Part B medical insurance. Regardless of age, if you have been receiving Social Security disability benefits for twenty-four months, you are eligible for Medicare. You may also be eligible if you have chronic kidney failure and require dialysis or kidney transplant.

If you are eligible, you are automatically covered. Hence there is no choice to make, but you will have to make choices about what kind of protection, if any, to buy to cover the substantial gaps that have appeared in Part A. Most categories of ordinary hospital costs are covered, but with limitations for each benefit period. A benefit period begins with admission to the hospital; you qualify for a new benefit period when you have been out of a hospital or skilled nursing facility for sixty days in a row. Although there are limits to the benefits available for each benefit period, there is no limit on the number of benefit periods you can have. All costs listed below are as of

Choosing a Health Insurance 45

1989—deductibles and copayments change each January 1. The hospital will bill Medicare for its part and will bill you for the deductible and copayments. The benefits under Part A include the following:

Hospital Care
Room and board in a semiprivate room.
Full coverage except for a $564 deductible.
All laboratory and X-ray charges.
All drugs provided by the hospital.
Blood transfusions after the third unit (pint). You must either pay for or replace the first three units.
Operating room and specialized unit charges (such as intensive-care unit, etc.).
All rehabilitation services, including physical therapy, occupational therapy, and speech therapy.

Skilled Nursing Facility
100 days per benefit period. You must have been in a hospital for at least three days within the month before admission to the skilled nursing facility. You must require skilled nursing care—this usually means dressing changes, complicated medication schedules, administration of frequent injections, use of and maintenance of various tubes, such as a gastrotomy feeding tube. Medicare will not pay for custodial nursing-home care.
First twenty days—full coverage.
Days twenty-one to 100—$65 per day copay.

Home Health Care
May provide skilled nursing care or physical, occupational, or speech therapy in certain cases. Does not cover full-time nursing care or custodial care.

Thus, Part A can leave you with significant out of pocket expenses. So you should consider buying one of the many policies sold to fill the Medicare gaps.

Part B, Medicare medical insurance benefits, can help pay for doctor's office visits, outpatient hospital care, various forms of therapy, home health care and equipment and supplies. If you are eligible for Medicare Part A, you are also eligible for Part B. To receive Part B benefits, you have to purchase the insurance by signing up during the three months before you turn sixty-five or during the first three months of any year thereafter.

The paying of bills under Part B (outpatient care) is, unfortunately, much more complicated then it is under Part A. Indeed you and your doctor will find your patience tested to the maximum over the EOB (Explanation of Benefits) with its awkward shape, microscopic print, and abbreviations, acronyms, and strange terminology. Even worse though is the failure even to receive the EOB, in which case no one gets paid, and confusion reigns.

It makes a difference if your doctor is a "participating" or "nonparticipating" doctor. Medicare pays benefits in either case, but the billing is somewhat different. If he is a participating doctor, he agrees to accept as payment in full the amount approved (which may be less than his usual fee), and he is paid directly (payment-to-the-doctor) by Medicare. He can bill you only for the difference between the amount actually paid by Medicare and the amount approved. Since Part B pays 80 percent of the approved amount after you have paid your yearly $75 deductible, the amount that your doctor can bill you for is 20 percent of the amount approved plus however much of the deductible you have not yet paid. But in no case will you be required to pay more than $1,370 per year for doctor bills.

If your doctor is a nonparticipating doctor, you submit your bill to Medicare, and you get the payment. You can either mail an itemized bill, or you can submit Part II of HCFA Form 1500; you must include your claim number (shown on your medical insurance card) with each claim. Medicare will pay you 80 percent of the amount approved, less whatever you may owe on the year's deductible. In the case of a nonparticipating doctor, the bill is usually greater than the amount approved. Even here, however, there are legislated and decreed rules that limit the amount that a doctor can legally charge you, even if he is a nonparticipating doctor.

The amount approved is sometimes called a reasonable charge. This suggests that a fee higher than the approved amount is unreasonable. And, indeed, it may be. On the other hand it may not be. From 1982 until January 1, 1987, Medicare payments to physicians were frozen by an act of Congress. It was literally against the law to charge more for a given service in 1986 than in 1982. Furthermore, the amount approved for all physicians' services was reduced by 1 percent in March 1986. Since the freeze ended there has been an upward adjustment of the approved amounts based on an incredibly complicated formula. Participating and nonparticipating doctors may be entitled to different payments by Medicare. The new rules are especially difficult for nonparticipating doctors, who cannot calculate their proper fee without data that Medicare has but will release only very reluctantly. There is thus great pressure to accept assignment.

Physicians' fees may be further restricted by the Medicare determination that a service was unnecessary. A variation of that is the decision that the level of service was inappropriate. Hospital visits, for example, are usually classified as brief, intermediate, extensive, etc. Your physician may bill for an intermediate hospital visit, but Medicare may decree that a brief hospital visit would have been sufficient and so allow only the lower fee that corresponds to a brief hospital visit.

All this gives doctors and their business managers great headaches, but does not directly involve you. But if the present trend continues so that doctors receive appreciably lower fees for service provided to Medicare patients than to fee-for-service patients, there may be problems ahead.

In any case, you do need to know that if your doctor is nonparticipating, you may be responsible for more than the "approved, or reasonable" amount.

The benefits covered by part B include the following:

Physician's services, in any location or facility, but excluding routine physicals and screening tests, cosmetic surgery, and mental illness fees in excess of $250 per year.
Pneumonia vaccine; other immunization not usually covered.
Laboratory services.
X rays.
Medical supplies, prescription drugs, electrocardiograms.
Physical and speech therapy.
Ambulance service when medically necessary.
Home health visits by an approved agency.

Thus, Part B is good medical insurance, very well worth the premium, even with the yearly $75 deductible. The lack of coverage for a routine physical is a theoretically important limitation but, by the time you are sixty-five, if you have no legitimate diagnosis to justify the examination, you really shouldn't complain!

As we have seen, there are significant out-of-pocket expenses for medical care under Medicare, so you should consider buying some supplementary insurance. There are many policies on the market, including some Blue Cross/Blue Shield plans. Another option that you may have is to join an HMO. Some geriatricians are recommending HMOs as a promising solution to the problem of fragmented, inefficient, and increasingly expensive care for the elderly. The Congress had endorsed this view through the passage of the Tax Equity and Fiscal Responsibility Act of 1982, which allows HMOs to contract with the Health Care Financing Administration (HCFA) to provide medical care for the elderly on a prospective, capitated basis. As of March 1, 1987, 3 percent of the Medicare population, or nearly 870,000 people, were enrolled in 151 HMOs in thirty-eight states (17).

If you do have the option of joining an HMO under Medicare, the issues are those we discussed in the section on HMOs. There is an additional concern, however. Older people need more medical, and especially hospital care, but HMOs survive by their ability to limit hospital costs. HMOs may "run the risk of losing vast amounts of money on the care of the elderly or exploiting this group for profit. Both of these possibilities have already occurred. . . ."(18) Two large HMOs dropped out of their contracts because of insufferable losses, and several Medicare HMOs in Florida "have been investigated for deceptive enrollment tactics, questionable medical care, and other abuses"(18). A report for the Senate Committee on Aging (17) found that "Health Care Finance Administration (HCFA) has relied too heavily on the HMOs to monitor and regulate themselves—creating an environment in which the Medicare beneficiary is highly exposed to crass and unethical marketing, substandard care, and unpredictable breaks in health insurance coverage."

So, if you are considering joining a Medicare-HMO plan, make sure it has a good history and is doing a good job taking care of Medicare patients.

If you are eligible for Medicaid, all the gaps in Medicare will be filled, and you will have no out-of-pocket expenses.

MEDICAID

Medicaid is a government program of medical assistance authorized by Title IX of the Social Security Act, signed into law by President Johnson on July 30, 1965. It provides for health care for some individuals who cannot otherwise afford it. It is a state program, but the federal government provides 50 to 80 percent of the program's costs, depending on the state's per-capita income. In order to qualify for federal funds, a state's Medicaid program must, at a minimum, cover the state's welfare population as well as those eligible for the federally funded program of assistance for the aged, blind, and disabled, and to families eligible for aid under the Aid to Families of Dependent Children program. A state may also choose to cover the "medically indigent"—those persons whose incomes are too high to qualify for welfare, but who find themselves faced with unmanageably high medical expenses.

The program must provide five basic services:

inpatient hospital services (excluding hospitals for mental illness)
outpatient hospital services
laboratory and X-ray services
skilled nursing-home services
physician's services.

States may choose to include other services, such as nonphysician medical care, home health services, dental services, drugs, dentures, prosthetic devices, and mental health services (inpatient or outpatient).

If you are eligible, you will usually be issued a Medicaid card to present to your doctor, therapist, pharmacist, or hospital. The cost of this medical care is paid for by general tax revenues. Any participating provider automatically agrees to accept as full payment the Medicaid allowance. The provider has to bill Medicaid; it is unlawful for the provider to bill or charge you in any way, except for the minimal copayment required by some programs.

The goal of the program is to provide medical care of high quality that will be readily available to those unable to pay for it. To help reach that goal, medical care providers are supposed to be paid usual and customary fees. In practice, however, Medicaid fees are often considerably below the prevailing rates in the community, payment is sometimes very late, and the billing process is complicated and costly. Consequently, the goal of participation by all physicians is rarely met, and patients often have to turn to large clinics or institutions to receive care. Nonetheless, if you are eligible, you can, with some perseverance, obtain adequate medical care that you might otherwise be unable to purchase.

CHOOSING A MEDICAL INSURANCE PLAN

It may be difficult to decide which of several insurance plans is best for you. The preceding material has highlighted several key issues for consideration, but here the salient points will be recapitulated.

You might start by trying to anticipate your need for medical services. While one can never predict a sudden illness or accident, many medical needs can be predicted. If you are relatively young (and I won't even attempt to define "young"), have excellent health, never go to doctors, and don't expect to, then your anticipated need for services is obviously minimal. If, on the other hand, you have a chronic condition that requires continuing medical services, such as diabetes with complications or symptomatic heart disease, then obviously you can anticipate considerable need for medical services. There are also less obvious aspects to the issue of medical needs. Even if you are young and healthy, if you believe in having periodic or routine examinations and tests such as complete physicals, mammography, PAP smears, and other aspects of preventive medicine, you have a significant demand for medical services. If you have babies who need frequent visits to the pediatrician, if a pregnancy is possible or likely, if you need a lot of medication (including birth-control pills), these factors may influence your choice of health insurance. So the first step is to consider carefully your own and your family's anticipated medical needs, including routine and preventive services, medications, and obstetric care. Include the possibility of a disastrous illness or injury or the need for long-term psychiatric hospitalization or treatment, an area often poorly covered.

Consider now the choice of health insurance based solely on cost. The cheapest is not necessarily the least costly. If you anticipate minimal medical needs, then you may well decide to choose the health insurance plan that has the lowest rates. Such a plan is likely to exclude coverage for preventive medicine and routine checkups. It is also likely not to have first-dollar coverage. It is likely to have cost-sharing features such as a yearly deductible, a copayment expense for each medical service, and a coinsurance feature such that you pay a portion of all the medical bills (usually 10–20 percent). But if you do not require many medical services, you will not have much cost to share, and so will come out ahead financially. Keep in mind, however, that if you have very little financial reserve, the cost-sharing expense of even a relatively minor illness can be demanding on your funds.

If you anticipate moderate health-care costs such as occasional physician office visits and perhaps one physical exam per year, plus occasional prescriptions, then deciding which insurance plan is most economical may be more difficult. Assuming that you have several plans to choose from, look at the one with the least expensive premium first. Consider what cost-sharing features there are, and what services are not covered at all. Then go back to your record of your anticipated medical needs for the year and estimate the out-of-pocket expenses. Add the out-of-pocket expenses to the premiums, and you have your anticipated medical costs. Compare this sum to the premium of a first-dollar, no-cost-sharing plan; this will indicate which plan is likely to be more economical for you.

If, finally, you anticipate the need for frequent medical services and continuing use of prescription medications, then you should choose the plan that has the most extensive coverage and the least cost sharing, even if the premiums are high.

So far we have been looking only at cost. But that may not be the sole, or even major, criterion by which you wish to choose your health-insurance plan. Perhaps the premiums are paid in whole or in part by your employer, or perhaps you have enough money to be able to afford the best, and are interested above all in the quality of health care. How, then, is one to choose? As we have seen, the data shows, contrary to the opinions of many, that there is no demonstrable, consistent difference in the quality of care between various forms of health insurance: conventional health insurance, HMOs (Health Maintenance Organizations), and PPOs (Preferred Provider Organizations). (This does not exclude the possibility that you have the choice of a particularly good plan, superior to any others available in your community.) But even if the quality of care is not demonstrably different, the quality of service may be. The choice here is partly a matter of personal preference.

Choosing a Health Insurance

Conventional health insurance, with basic benefits and major medical coverage, offers almost no restrictions on choice of physicians, hospitals, location, or kind of treatment. You can change doctors at will, you can see multiple doctors sequentially or simultaneously, if that is your wish. You can decide which hospital to use for what illness. You can go see a specialist without a referral, and you can go to an emergency room. But it is also up to you to find a doctor or other medical care provider, and it is up to you to assess the quality of care you receive. And it is up to you to pay the cost sharing and the services not covered, which may include office visits and preventive health care.

Conventional health insurance is a way of paying for medical care; the insurance company is a fiscal intermediary and does not affect the practice of medicine. In contrast to this, the alternative insurances are so-called managed-care plans. These include HMOs and PPOs. Although there are significant differences between the varieties of HMOs and PPOs, they share certain features in common. All seek active influence over the practice of medicine. The chief issue is cost. Physicians are provided with strong (financial) incentives to minimize the cost of care. Medical costs are further contained by restricting your choice of physicians to those who practice by the rules of the plan and by limiting your access to consultants. You will usually have to obtain a referral from your primary-care physician if you want to see a consultant or a subspecialist.

Cost is not the only element monitored; to a varying degree the quality of care is also monitored. Substandard practices are identified and corrected. Furthermore, the qualifications of participating physicians are screened, and each physician's work is subject to the scrutiny of his peers.

HMOs offer you the advantage of organized, coordinated, one-stop medical care, with first-dollar coverage, including checkups, preventive services, and health education. The disadvantage is that you have to use only the HMO's staff and facilities. Large HMOs provide a wide range of facilities and staff, but may have an impersonal, institutional quality. This is especially true for staff model HMOs, in which the doctors are all salaried and see only HMO patients. Group practice HMOs and, even more so, IPA (Independent Practice Association) HMOs have some of the practice style characteristics of ordinary fee-for-service medical care, but give up some of the benefits that derive from the more tightly organized staff-model HMOs.

PPOs are often described as intermediate plans between conventional health insurance and HMOs. Physicians have strong financial incentives to minimize services, consultations, and overall cost of care, but they are paid on a fee-for-service basis and control their own individual offices and practice style. For the patient there is still the same trade-off: less expensive health insurance for the price of some restriction of access to physicians, hospitals and other health-care providers.

Table 1 which follows summarizes some of the features of PPOs, HMOs, and Conventional health insurance.

TABLE 1.

	Conventional Insurance	HMO	PPO
Hospital Costs	Fully covered basic benefit, usually 60–365 days. Cost sharing features usual.	Fully covered	Fully covered
Surgical Fees	Part of basic benefit. Pays according to fee schedule—may not pay full cost.	Fully covered.	Fully covered if surgeon is a preferred provider. Cost sharing if out of network.
Office Visits	Covered if policy includes Major Medical benefits. Cost-sharing usual.	Fully covered.	Fully covered for preferred provider. Cost sharing if out of network.
Mental Health	Very limited for both in- and outpatient care.	Same as conventional insurance. May include limited chemical dependency services.	Same as HMO.
Catastrophic Illness	Not usually covered. May be an option for additional premium.	Usually covered—HMO contracts with conventional insurance company.	Same as conventional insurance.
Other Benefits*	Very variable. Some policies are very limited.	Very rich benefit package if federally qualified; otherwise variable.	Usually intermediate between conventional insurance and HMO.
Freedom of Choice	Unrestricted choice of MD, hospital or geographic location of services.	Most restricted. You must use HMO MDs, facilities and hospitals. Coverage outside of geographic area in emergency only.	More restricted than conventional insurance but less than HMOs

* = Preventive services, checkups, health education, dietary services, prostheses, equipment such as blood sugar monitors, home care.

Access to Consultants	Unlimited.	Restricted to HMO consultants. You may need referral from primary care MD.	Usually need referral from primary care MD. Greater selection (usually) than HMO. Full coverage only for network consultant.
Practice Style	Not affected by insurance. Depends on MD and practice setting that you choose.	Variable. Staff-model HMO is highly organized, centralized and may be impersonal. IPA model is more like private practice. Group practice model is intermediate.	Resembles private practice but there are controls and restrictions placed on primary care MDs.
Cost Sharing	Deductible, co-payment and co-insurance is common.	None, or minimal co-payment. "First dollar" coverage is the rule.	More cost sharing than HMO, less than conventional insurance.
Making Claims	A claim form must be filed for each service. Either you do it, and pay the MD directly, or he does it and bills you for the difference. The hospital bills the insurance company directly.	No claim forms, no paper work for you, unless you apply for reimbursement for out-of-area services. You never see a bill.	The preferred provider bills the PPO; no paper work for you. If you go out of network, you may have to pay the MD and file for reimbursement.
Premiums	Very variable. Lowest premiums for plans with large cost sharing and restricted services.	Very variable. Tend toward the high side.	Very variable. Often intermediated between HMO and conventional insurance.
Medication	Often not covered; may be extra charge option.	Often covered, usually with small co-payment. Some restrictions on drugs and pharmacies.	Same as HMO.

3

MEDICAL TESTS
Kurt Link, M.D.

If you get medical care for any but the simplest ailments, you will be subjected to medical tests. Modern medical tests allow a precision of diagnosis undreamed of by clinicians of even fifty years ago. The application of modern physics, automation, electronics, computer science, mathematics, and biochemistry to clinical medicine makes it possible for your doctors to see your every organ and the structures within them, to measure, monitor and analyze the electrical forces of your brain, heart, and nerves, to measure the minutest fluctuation in your body chemistry, to measure the concentration of the myriad of hormones in your body, even those present in trace amounts, to measure how much blood your heart is pumping per beat or per minute, and how much blood is flowing to your vital organs. These tests are an essential part of the dramatic successes of modern medicine. But medical tests can be an expensive, complicated, and even dangerous business; their proper use is art as well as science and can tax the skill of the most experienced clinician.

SELECTING AND INTERPRETING TESTS

Test results are not black or white. There are shades of gray; there is ambiguity. This applies even to a concept so basic as the definition of "normal." For many tests, defining what is normal is a problem because there is a large range of values, all of which are normal. There is no clear marker of the place where the extreme of normal ends and the truly abnormal begins. It is like trying to define abnormalities of body height. Suppose you are interested in growth disturbances and want to study individuals who are abnormally short or abnormally tall. Three feet tall or even four feet tall for an adult is abnormally small. Five-foot-two is not abnormal. Where is one to

Medical Tests

draw the line? In fact, even four feet tall may be normal for some ethnic groups, and one look at the suits of armor of medieval times will tell you that today's "normal" height is unlike yesterday's. Furthermore, normal for men is different from normal for women. Similar considerations apply to tall stature.

Like bodily stature, many common medical measurements show this kind of continuous range of values. In these cases a normal range is defined by looking at the spread of values of a random or supposedly normal population, and taking the middle 90 percent as the normal range. Statisticians define this range as the median plus-or-minus two standard deviations. In height for example, we might say that anyone who is shorter than 95 percent of the general population, or is taller than 95 percent of the population, is abnormal with respect to height.

Normal values for the blood concentration of sodium, potassium, hemoglobin, and many other measurements are, in fact, defined in this way. Thus, for this kind of test 10 percent of healthy individuals will by definition, have results outside the normal range.

One could of course eliminate the category of the healthy individual with an abnormal result by raising the upper limit of normal so high (say 7 feet tall) that virtually everyone with a value greater than that would be truly abnormal. But since these continuously variable measurements have an overlap between normal and abnormal individuals, setting the limits too high will fail to detect mildly abnormal conditions (i.e., 6 feet, 11 inches). The 90 percent cutoff, it turns out, is often the best discriminator: It doesn't label many normal individuals as abnormal, and it doesn't fail to diagnose most abnormal individuals.

But this leaves us with the problem of deciding if the abnormal test result really means that you are abnormal and, if so, what to do about it. If the upper limit of normal for serum sodium concentration is 145 (milliequivalent per liter), and your result comes back 146, the usual computer-generated report will flag this value as abnormal by an asterisk, bold-faced type, red ink, etc. If this occurs in the context of a routine checkup, and there appears to be nothing the matter with you, your doctor will probably and properly ignore the test result, assuming that it is a lab error or that you are in that 5 percent of healthy individuals with an "abnormally" high serum sodium concentration. He will also hope that you are not going to ask to see a copy of the actual laboratory report for fear of having a lot of explaining to do. If the same 146 value occurred while you were in the hospital and surviving on intravenous fluids, your doctor's response might be different. In that context, for example, an adjustment of the concentration of your IV fluids might be in order, or the test might be repeated to double-check its accuracy.

There are other problems with the 90 percent cutoff. It assumes that the general population upon which the normal range is based is, in fact, normal. But if 60 percent of the population is abnormal, it will not do to define normal as the mean +/− 2 standard deviations.

Cholesterol testing provides an example. It turns out that what was normal in 1987 is now considered too high. What we were accepting as the upper limit of normal based on the mean +/− 2 SD (standard deviations) is associated with considerable risk for heart attacks. So now we have a lower upper limit of normal for cholesterol. "Normal," in this context may be defined as the value associated with the absence of disease or illness.

Of course not all medical measurements are a matter of degree. Pregnancy tests are usually considered as positive or negative. There are tests for mononucleosis, syphilis, and many other conditions in this category. But even in the case of a positive pregnancy test, interpretation of the test is still required. A positive test is assumed to mean that the patient has a normal pregnancy. But a tubal pregnancy will also give a positive test, and so will certain tumors. So even pregnancy testing is not really a simple yes-or-no affair.

There are, of course, other kinds of problems in the interpretation of tests. No medical test is 100 percent accurate. There are false positive and false negative results. A false positive result occurs when the test is positive for a condition but you don't have it. And a false negative occurs when you do have the condition being tested for, but the test is negative.

We will discuss the implications of these false positive and negative results below. For the moment I would note only that it is important, when choosing a test, to be aware of the false positive/negative rates and be prepared to confirm the result of the test, especially if it does not fit the overall clinical picture. If for, example, your blood count shows a severe anemia, but you are feeling perfectly well, you might suspect that there is a problem with the test and not with your health. If, on the other hand you have a sore throat, fever, swollen glands, rash, and all other signs and symptoms of mononucleosis, but the test is negative, perhaps the test should be repeated before diagnosis of mononucleosis is abandoned.

False positive and false negative results are inherent in the tests; they occur even when the test is properly done. If the test is done improperly, of course, or if the specimen or report or film is labeled with someone else's name, or the sample has been stored improperly before being processed, or if some other technical error occurs, then the results may be wrong on that account. A good laboratory can minimize but never completely eliminate these problems. When the result of a test is a complete surprise to the doctor or the result just doesn't fit, he should suspect lab error.

The proper interpretation of test results requires familiarity with the disease being tested for. For example, in the case of mononucleosis, it is important to know that it may take days or even weeks for the test to turn positive. Other aspects of testing have to be taken into account. To interpret the result of a test of your blood sugar properly, it is important to know when you last ate. Thyroid tests will be affected if you are taking birth-control pills, and tests that indicate the presence of hepatitis may be due to drinking too much alcohol. Sometimes one disease will affect the results of tests for another. Suppose, for example, you are going to have a lung scan because of a suspicion that you may have a blood clot in your lungs; if you have emphysema or bronchitis, your lung scan may be abnormal even if you don't have a blood clot.

In short, selecting the proper test can be a test of your clinician's skills. He must understand the disease, the test, and your particular case. The test must be on target; it must be suited for the purpose to which it is put; it must provide information that will make a difference; it must be available and affordable; it must be carried out properly.

Let us look at these points one by one. The test must be on target. If you have a stomachache because you are depressed, X rays of your stomach will not be helpful, no matter how skillfully done. And if you are depressed because your thyroid gland is not working, no psychotherapy or antidepressant will make you feel better.

A test should be suited to its purpose. Tests can be performed for a variety of reasons. A test that is good for diagnosis when you are ill may not be good for screening purposes when you are well. So the proper choice of a test will depend in part on the purpose of the tests.

The test must provide information that will make a difference. If the result will not change the diagnosis, lead to a change in therapy, or indicate prognosis or provide some other useful information, why bother doing it?

Some practical issues also arise. Your clinician must know what tests exist and also what tests are available in your community. Some esoteric test may not be available, or if available, done so infrequently or so inexpertly as to make the result unreliable. Cost factors exist too. Is it worth $300 to find a hairline stress fracture in your foot with a bone scan, or should you just assume that it might be there and stop running for a few weeks?

Knowing the benefits of a test is not enough. The risk of a test must also be taken into account. As in the case of selecting a medication, or in choosing any kind of therapy or medical intervention, the potential benefit must be weighed against the risk. And all tests have risks.

Some tests are risky in the performing. Tests that require the insertion of needles or catheters, or require the injection of dyes, or exposure to radiation, or insertion of tubes into orifices—all these have risks of injury from the test procedure. Some tests are virtually harmless in this regard: taking a blood sample from the finger or a vein, a sonogram, a chest X ray, a urinalysis.

But harmless tests can have risks too. A false positive test can cause harm. Suppose your chest X ray shows a shadow suspicious for lung cancer. The next step may be a relatively harmless CAT scan of the chest and examination of the sputum. Unfortunately, if these are negative, the possibility of a cancer is still not ruled out. So your doctor recommends a bronchoscopy; he looks into your windpipe and bronchial tubes with a flexible tube to see the problem directly. But it may be too deep in the lung to be seen. The only way to settle the issue, finally, is to do chest surgery and a biopsy. Peril accompanies you on every step of this unhappy path; if you are fortunate and experience no complications, you will suffer only pain and expense to find out that the shadow was just a false positive—scar tissue from a long-ago infection.

A false positive test for AIDS may destroy your peace of mind and sex life; if you are a pilot, a false positive EKG may jeopardize your job; a false positive PAP smear may lead to surgery.

A false negative test can be just as harmful. If a biopsy fails to show the presence of a malignancy, a chance at cure may be missed. If a lung scan fails to show the first blood clot in your lung, the second may prove fatal.

Even a true positive or true negative test result can cause problems. Suppose your doctor, hearing a "click" when listening to your heart, orders an echocardiogram, which shows that you have a harmless variety of the heart condition known as mitral prolapse. You run to the books, discover that mitral prolapse can be associated with sudden death or with infections on the mitral heart valve. Before long you are filled with dread, you develop palpitations and chest pains. Your physician's assurance that these complications do not occur in cases such as yours only fuel your paranoia, and you begin to seek multiple medical opinions. Meanwhile you are denied life insurance, and you begin to fear for your life. By this time you (and your doctor) will wish that the echocardiogram that proved positive had never been done.

What about the true negative? Suppose you smoke cigarettes. You begin to worry about having lung cancer. You ask for a chest X ray. Your doctor orders it, and it is a true negative. With a sigh of relief, you open a new pack of cigarettes, secure in the knowledge that you don't have cancer.

So before you take a test you should have confidence that the test is appropriate and that the benefits outweigh the risks. If you know that routine chest X rays have a relatively high risk of false positive results and that the benefits of a true positive are limited by the very low cure rate for lung cancers detected in this way, you may choose to spend your X ray money on a new pair of shoes (and hopefully give up smoking before anything shows up).

WHY TEST AND WHEN?

Tests serve various purposes. Tests may be used to screen for unsuspected conditions when you are feeling well, to make a diagnosis when you are feeling ill, to monitor the progress of your illness after a diagnosis has been made, to guide or monitor therapy when you are under treatment. These are the usual clinical purposes of tests. Medical tests are also used as tools of law enforcement or social policy as in mandatory drug screening and testing for conditions that cause concern to society such as AIDS and other sexually transmittable diseases. Each of these purposes require different kinds of tests, so the proper selection of a test depends in part on defining precisely the goal in mind.

Why would you subject yourself to a medical test (known as a screening test) when you are feeling well? The answer is simple: to detect a problem at the earliest possible stage, before you have symptoms, so that treatment can cure the problem or prevent complications. But if this sounds simple, its application is not.

The first issue is what diseases or conditions to test for. There is no point or, at least, little point to screening for conditions that require no treatment or are minor in nature. Why screen for psoriasis or flat feet? If the condition is not bothering you, why bother it? Nor is there much point to screening for untreatable or incurable disease. Multiple sclerosis is a neurologic disease for which no effective treatment exists. If you had the condition and it could be detected before you had any symptoms, its discovery would not help you and might harm you psychologically. The only reason to test in cases like these are when the disease is communicable (such as asymptomatic venereal disease) and there are thus public-health reasons to screen, or if the disease is hereditary. But in general, screening should be directed at important conditions for which effective treatment exists.

However, there is not much point in screening for rare diseases either. The yield of cases found will be small, the cost per case found will be great, and the problem of false positives will be large. This last point is somewhat technical but important. If a test has a low false-positive rate such as 1 per 1,000, you might assume that the false-positive problem will be small. But if the disease being tested for is rare, occurring, for example, in 1 per 10,000 of the population being tested, then for every 10,000 persons tested, there will be ten false-positive tests and only one true positive. So if you test positive with the "good" test, the chances are still 10 out of 11 that you *don't* have the disease. Only if the rare disease occurs frequently in a particular population, could screening those persons prove helpful. Testing the general population for a rare disease is not a good idea.

Finding a disease before it causes symptoms is valuable only if treatment is more effective in the presymptomatic phase. High blood pressure is the classic example. Treatment before symptoms occur prevents strokes; if you wait until there are symptoms, treatment may come too late. Breast cancers caught early are more likely to be cured, so screening for breast cancer is useful. But if you have a lung cancer discovered by routine chest X ray, you will not fare any better than if it was discovered after you have symptoms, which is why the routine chest X ray has fallen out of favor.

Consider now the test itself. An important factor is the accuracy of the test. You do not want a test with a large false-positive rate when testing a large asymptomatic population. A high false-positive rate often means high costs and hazards of confirmatory and follow-up testing. Sometimes the screening does more harm than good. It has been argued, for example, that this is true in the case of testing the stool for traces of blood to detect early bowel cancer (1). A positive test implies follow-up tests, usually including colonoscopy. The cost, discomfort, and hazard of that procedure may outweigh the benefit of finding a few unsuspected cases of bowel cancer. False negative results on the other hand may cause a dangerous delay in diagnosis.

Cost is always a factor, but especially so for screening tests, at least when viewed from the public-health perspective. If you have to screen a thousand persons to find one case, that find costs a thousand times the cost of each test. Since the resources available for medical care are limited, you always have to ask if this kind of screening test is the best use of limited health-care dollars.

A screening test must be readily available and safe and acceptable to persons who are feeling well. You may not wish to subject yourself to a dangerous or painful test if you are feeling fine.

To summarize: Screening tests should test for common, important diseases that are treatable. Treatment in the presymptomatic phase should be more efficacious than in the symptomatic phase. The test should have a low false-positive rate, be relatively inexpensive, harmless, and painless. As we shall see in the chapter on staying healthy, the number of such tests is surprisingly small.

Consider now a test to diagnose a condition when you are sick. After you have described all your symptoms and the circumstances of your malady, your doctor will examine you, and then, you hope, he will have narrowed the possibilities down to a few considerations, or will at least have an idea of what kind of ailment you have. He may decide that you have an infection or some kind of heart trouble, etc. Now you want a test that has a low false-negative rate. If the test is negative you want to be sure that means you really don't have the disease, in spite of the clinical suspicion that you do. A test that is expensive or painful or even dangerous may be acceptable now, because there *is* an illness at hand, and an accurate diagnosis is important.

Another use of tests is to monitor the progress of disease. In this case the diagnosis—hepatitis, for example—is known. You want to be tested periodically to monitor the progress of your disease. Such a test, since it will be done repeatedly, must not be hazardous or very painful, and the cost must be at least reasonable. The test need not be unique to your condition, but it does need to be a sensitive indicator of how you are faring. The SGOT (serum glutamic-oxaloacetic transaminase, a test for damage to hepatic cells) is abnormal in many diverse conditions— abnormality is not in any way proof of hepatitis—but it is always abnormal in hepatitis and is a very sensitive indicator of the condition's severity, so it is a good test to monitor if the diagnosis has been proved in other ways.

Finally, consider tests to monitor your therapy. If you are taking a potentially toxic drug (virtually any drug), it may be possible to test periodically for the earliest signs of such toxicity. Some diuretic fluid pills, for example, cause a loss of vital potassium. It is common practice to check the potassium level in the blood to detect this problem early. Another kind of test used to guide therapy is the measurement of the amount of drug in your blood. In this case precision is vital. If you have diabetes, it makes little difference if your blood sugar at any moment is 245 or 260 (milligrams per decaliter). But if you are taking the heart medicine digoxin, the precision of the measurement is crucial. The concentration of digoxin in the blood is minute; the slightest variation has significance. The test will be worthless if it is not highly precise.

I will not attempt to deal here with use of tests to detect illegal drug usage or mandatory testing for AIDS or other conditions that are a threat to society. I would note, however, that the complexities of test selection and interpretation apply in this context just as they do in the clinical context. Legislators need to deal adequately with these issues if their rules and laws are to be fair and effective.

COMMONLY USED TESTS

Having reviewed some aspects of the interpretation and selection of medical tests, let us now consider some commonly used tests.

Imaging

Superman's X ray vision has nothing over today's radiologist's vision.

He has more than X-ray vision; he has computerized vision, magnetic resonance vision, sonographic vision, and nuclear vision.

X Ray. The ordinary X ray is no longer a marvel; it is your old-fashioned, low-tech, traditional form of imaging. But it is still valuable and much used. Its history is steeped in myth and heroism. The early practitioners, ignorant of its potentially destructive force, lost their fingers to the damaging X rays and developed leukemia and all kinds of cancers. But today's X ray is performed with machines that emit a highly controlled, highly directed, very limited energy, which produces images of great detail. The theoretical hazard of an ordinary X ray is immeasurably small. If there is even a slight possibility that an X ray will produce useful information about your case, the benefit is sure to outweigh the risk.

Ordinary X rays are the standard for detecting fractures and many other abnormalities of bone. The chest X ray detects pneumonia, collapsed lung, and abnormalities of the size or shape of the heart and aorta. A plain X ray of the abdomen can sometimes detect bowel obstruction or perforated ulcer.

A bit more complex is the use of barium or dyes to improve the images obtained with ordinary X rays. When the old-time radio character, the invisible Shadow, was catching crooks, his more savvy enemies would detect his presence by blowing smoke into the room. In the same way, putting barium into your stomach or colon may reveal details of these organs not otherwise visible by ordinary X rays. Hence the upper GI (gastrointestinal) series, in which you swallow barium that outlines the esophagus, stomach, and duodenum to reveal tumors, scar tissue, or ulcers. Hence too, the barium enema, in which the barium is poured into the colon via an enema, to reveal cancers, diverticulitis, or inflammation (ulcerative colitis, Crohn disease).

The IVP is a different kind of dye test. The kidneys do not show up very well with ordinary X rays. But if a dye that is concentrated by the kidneys is injected intravenously, a very detailed image is produced. This test is called an intravenous pyelogram or IVP. One problem with this test is the fairly frequent occurrence of allergic or other adverse reactions to the dye. Recently a so-called nonionic dye has been developed. This dye causes far fewer adverse reactions but is enormously expensive. This situation has sparked a lively debate because the reactions are sometimes serious, but the cost of using only the new dye would run into millions yearly. The medical, legal, and ethical ramifications are fascinating, but not entirely pertinent here. In any case, the IVP can be further refined by obtaining special X rays that show a picture of just a thin slice, known as a tomogram, of the kidney. This X ray is a nephrotomogram. In tests of the kidney, that wonderful organ is variously referred to as kidney, nephron, pyelo, or renal, as in kidney biopsy, renal scan, intravenous pyelogram, nephrotomogram. Perhaps the inventor of each test was proficient in a different language, so we have Greek, Latin, and Anglo-Saxon terms all mixed up.

Mammography. Another test done with X rays. Breast cancers too small to feel can sometimes be detected by telltale calcium deposits detectable with the special X ray technique used in mammography. At one time there was concern about the exposure to X ray, especially since mammography is likely to be done many times in a woman's life span. But newer machines have reduced the radiation risk to the vanishing point, while increasing experience with the technique has led to ever more precise diagnoses.

Angiograph. Another form of X ray in which dye is used to show up structures that would otherwise be invisible. In this case the dye is injected into the blood vessels of the diseased organ. A cerebral angiogram, for example, may show the cluster of abnormal blood vessels that indicates the presence of a brain cancer. A blockage of the arteries in the brain may explain a stroke. An angiogram of the kidney arteries may pinpoint the cause of your high blood pressure.

Angiography may be a difficult test to perform. The angiographer—often a radiologist with special skills—must be able to thread a tube from its point of entry through your skin (usually near the elbow or the groin) through your arteries until it reaches its destination, which may be your neck or heart or interior. The dye has to be injected under pressure—usually by machine—and this can further injure an already damaged organ. Angiography is an example of a so-called invasive test—in which the interior of the body is invaded; such tests all have risk of causing damage, and so their use must be carefully considered.

CAT Scan. Ordinary X ray images depend on the fact that some tissues block X rays more than others. Bones stop X rays cold, so they show up very well. Air lets X rays through, so it too shows up well. But if two adjacent tissues absorb X rays almost equally well, the border between them may not be detectable with ordinary X rays. This problem can be partly overcome by use of the CAT (computerized axial tomography) scan. The image is obtained through the use of ordinary X rays but the energy of the X rays is not captured by film. It is, instead, fed to a computer, which then generates the image. The computer receives data as the X-ray tube rotates 360 degrees around the part being scanned. The data for a infinite number of potential images is stored. The radiologist then has the computer construct whatever single image or view he wants to look at. He can enlarge or diminish, enhance or dim any component of the image. He can literally turn the image this way and that on the computer screen. The CAT scanner is a multimillion dollar machine, but it is worth every penny.

MRI. There are clinical uses for non-X-ray images too. The MRI (Magnetic Resonance Imager) produces images using magnetic fields and radio-frequency energy. Even with the CAT scan, the details of X-ray images depend on the ease with which X rays can penetrate various tissues. If different parts of the brain let X rays penetrate to the same extent, those parts will not be distinguishable one from the other; it is like trying to see a sheet of glass immersed in water. The MRI, however, distinguishes among various tissues by differences in their chemical makeup. So it can distinguish details not visible by X-ray images. The MRI is an enormous and enormously expensive machine. To have your image made, you are placed on a table that slides into a chamber within the machine. Once inside the MRI scanner, you are subjected to a powerful magnetic field, which lines up the nuclei of some of the hydrogen atoms of the part being imaged, like flags in a strong wind. You cannot take this test if you have any metal objects in your body, or a pacemaker. With your hydrogen atoms thus at attention, you are zapped with a burst of radio-frequency energy. You feel none of this, but the proper radio-frequency pulse alters the energy level of some of the atoms (a condition known as resonance) and knocks them out of alignment. As soon as this pulse is over, the atoms rotate back into their previous position in the magnetic field. As they do so, they generate their own radio-frequency energy. It is this energy that is used to produce the final image. And what an image it is! Since each body tissue or structure has a different composition with respect to hydrogen, each creates a unique magnetic resonance pattern. Subtle differences in tissues can therefore be detected. Before MRI, only a surgeon at the operating table or a pathologist at the autopsy table ever saw such detail. The radiologist has become an anatomist, seeing the inner structure of your brain, the contents of your eyeball, and the nerve that leaves your spinal cord as it wends its way between your vertebrae.

Ultrasound is yet another form of energy that can be used to make an image. Inaudible, ultra-high-frequency "sounds" are directed against the part being examined. The waves that bounce back, the echoes, are recorded to produce the image. Unlike the CAT scan or MRI scan, the ultrasound image is not an immediately recognizable picture; it is a pie-shaped wedge of black and white patterns in which the outlines of the internal organs are recognizable only to a knowledgeable eye. But the ultrasound is easy to use (once you know how), the device is small enough to be portable, and its use is inexpensive and harmless. It can be used to study parts in motion such as the valves in the interior of the heart. It is safe enough to use in pregnant women. Indeed, it is *the* way to diagnose twin pregnancy. Ultrasound can detect fibroid tumors, ovarian cysts, and other gynecologic conditions. It is the best way to find gallstones. Urologists are even using an ultrasound device that can be inserted into the rectum to "see" the prostate gland.

Radioactive Imagings. The last imaging method, which is more than an imaging method, requires the use of radioactive materials. If you ingest radioactive technetium, for example, your thyroid gland will quickly capture it. The radiation emitted by your "hot" gland can then be used to form an image. There are many clinically useful radioactive compounds that will concentrate in various tissues and organs, such as damaged areas of the heart, fractures, cancers of bone, the lung, stomach cells, and others. The image is obtained by scanning the appropriate organ for radioactivity. These images are not of high quality or rich in detail, but imaging is only part of the value of the scans. Most nuclear scans provide an indication of the function of the tissue or organ being examined. In the case of the thyroid, for example, the extent to which the gland concentrates the radioactive isotope reflects the activity of the gland. A radioactive lung scan is commonly used to detect blood clots. A positive scan is caused by obstruction of blood flow to a portion of the lung. It is this functional impairment that is "seen," not a picture of the blood clot. A bone scan is not actually a picture of the bone; instead, it shows areas of bone that have an altered metabolism.

The disadvantage of nuclear scans is that they use dangerous radioactive compounds. The amount used is so small that no harm is done, but even so, pregnant women and children should not, as a rule, have nuclear scans. Besides their potential danger, nuclear scans are generally expensive and sometimes take hours to perform.

Electrical recordings.

Many of your body's activities produce electrical currents. In some cases recording and analyzing these currents can provide information about your bodily function or the presence of disease.

Electrocardiogram. Perhaps most familiar is the electrocardiogram. The electrocardiogram is a recording of the electrical activity of the heart. The first recording of the heart's electrical activity was accomplished more than a hundred years ago, by Augustus Waller. But it is the name of Willem Einthoven that is usually associated with the origins of electrocardiography. He won the 1924 Nobel Prize for his work, including his 1903 paper (2), in which he described the *elektrokardiogramm,* hence the usual abbreviation EKG. The old-time electrocardiographers could infer all kinds of noncardiac conditions from the EKG. They detected abnormalities of bodily chemistry, brain function, even glandular secretion. They read EKGs the way a seer reads tea leaves. But modern laboratory methods have, to some extent, done to EKGs what the pocket calculator has done to the slide rule. But the EKG is still of great value, especially for the diagnosis of heart attacks and irregularities of heart rhythm.

If your doctor suspects that you have an occasional or intermittent rhythm disturbance, he may have you wear a portable EKG monitor, the Holter monitor. This makes a record of every heartbeat for the duration of the monitoring period, usually twenty-four hours. A computer then scans the tracing of the approximately 100,000 heartbeats, detecting any abnormalities of rhythm. Irregular portions of the tracing can be displayed on an oscilloscope or printed on paper to facilitate analysis.

Electroencephalograms. (EEGs) are recordings of the electrical activity of your brain—your "brain waves." The recording is made by pasting to your scalp numerous small electrodes wired to the EEG machine. Sometimes parts of your scalp need to be shaved. Some EEG labs use electrodes in the form of small needles that the technician sticks into your scalp. Your brain waves show if you are awake or how deep in sleep you are, or if you are alive at all. EEG is crucial in the diagnosis of seizures or epilepsy and many other brain conditions.

Electromyograms. (EMGs) record the electrical activity of your nerves and muscles. Every time one of your nerves transmits a message, it produces electrical activity. The type of electrical wave, and its speed of travel, reveals much about the nerve's condition. Similarly, when a muscle contracts, it produces electrical activity in characteristic patterns both in health and disease. The EMG is a record of these electrical impulses. The EMG requires the insertion of small needles through the skin, and sometimes requires the neurologist doing the test to administer small electric shocks to see how your neuromuscular system responds.

Endoscopy.

Fiberoptic endoscopes have made it possible to peer into virtually every natural, and some unnatural, orifices of the human body. This ability to see directly into various organs sometimes allows an early diagnosis without the expense, delay, and uncertainty of conventional tests. The endoscopist can even at times do biopsies and limited surgery, such as removal of a polyp. Except for screening sigmoidoscopy (examination of the colon), most endoscopic procedures require extensive training, and are done by subspecialists.

Bronchoscopy is the examination of the bronchial tubes. After spraying the back of your throat with a local anesthetic, your doctor passes the bronchoscope through your mouth and down into your windpipe and then into the progressively smaller branches of your bronchial tree. He can see the condition of these delicate tubes and can use a tiny brush to rub some cells off the lining so that they can be examined in the laboratory. He can even pass a diminutive biopsy forceps out into the lung itself. A lung biopsy obtained in this way can sometimes replace an open lung biopsy, which requires the chest to be cut open. Bronchoscopy is most often recommended if there is a suspicion that you may have lung cancer, or if you are coughing up blood.

Upper gastrointestinal endoscopy is the examination of the esophagus, stomach, and possibly the duodenum just beyond the stomach. Endoscopy may be the best and fastest way to find the cause of internal bleeding, disease of the esophagus or stomach or duodenal ulcer. If internal bleeding is due to gastritis, the whole stomach lining may be weeping blood. In the case of an ulcer, the characteristic sore may be obvious, but a small stomach ulcer may be hidden in the stomach lining folds, like a tick hidden on the brow of a bulldog. Cancer, bleeding veins, and many other diseases of the upper tract may be diagnosed by endoscopy.

Sigmoidoscopy (from the Greek letter *sigma* or S) is examination of the lowest portion of the colon, which is S-shaped. Examinations used to be done with a sigmoidoscope that was straight, rigid, and hollow. Nowadays a flexible fiberoptic scope is commonly used. Sigmoidoscopy is often done as part of a cancer-screening examination. You lie on your side as the doctor passes the scope into the rectal opening. While he is engrossed in directing the scope around the partitions of the winding pink tunnel that is your colon, you will experience only a sense of pressure, bloating, and gas cramps. The examination takes about fifteen minutes and is usually done by a gastroenenterologist or primary-care physician.

Colonoscopy is more complete examination of the entire colon done with the much longer colonoscope. Colonoscopy takes special training; most often the test will be done by a gastroenterologist. You will be medicated to relax you and relieve any pain or spasm. The room is usually darkened. To see exactly where the end of the scope is, your doctor may from time to time push the tip toward your skin and see where the light glows from within your abdomen.

Colonoscopy is done to find and remove polyps or find the cause of rectal bleeding, such as tumors, diverticulitis, or inflammation.

Cystoscopy is the examination of the bladder. As you lie on the examining table with your legs apart and your feet up, the urologist passes the cystoscope into the urethral opening and on into the bladder where, with the aid of mirrors, he is able to look all around that roomy high-domed chamber. This examination is especially useful in the detection of bladder tumors or finding the source of blood in the urine.

Arthroscopy allows your orthopedist to see into the strange bloodless world of the joint cavities, lined with white glistening cartilage. Torn ligaments can be repaired, cartilage fragments removed, and rough surfaces sanded smooth.

There are other endoscopic tests, including those that look into the cavities of the nasal passages and larynx, the inside of the abdominal cavity, and the pelvic organs.

Blood Tests

There is little danger to having these tests, although they may leave a black-and-blue swelling. Rarely more serious complications occur—such as an infection or inflammation of the vein—especially in patients who have had surgery to remove the lymph glands from the armpit as in some operations for breast cancer. Or, if you have a tendency to bleed easily, there may be some bleeding, especially if an artery is punctured instead of a vein. Finally, some people faint when having blood drawn; a fall and injury can ensue.

Blood can be tested for the condition of the blood itself. Is there anemia, a problem with the white blood cells, or with the clotting mechanism? Or blood can be tested to determine its chemical composition. A common blood test is the biochemical profile known as the SMA 12 (named after the machine that can run twelve tests on one sample of blood). This test includes measurement of calcium, potassium, sodium and other minerals, sugar, cholesterol and other blood fats, and BUN and creatinine which are waste products excreted by the kidney.

It is now possible, using sophisticated radioactively labeled reagents, to measure the extremely minute concentrations of various hormones in the blood, including the hormones secreted by the thyroid gland, the ovaries and testes, the pituitary, the pancreas, the parathyroid, and the adrenal glands. These measurements, known as radioimmunoassays, have taught researchers much about the function of these glands, and have greatly aided clinicians in the diagnosis of disorders of the endocrine system.

Many infections can be detected by measuring the antibodies in your blood. If you are making an antibody against an infectious agent, that means you must at some time have come in contact with that agent. Sometimes that is all that can be said, but if serial measurements show a rise of antibody level, then you have proof positive that there has been a recent infection. Antibody tests can also tell if you are immune to certain infections or if you are susceptible to infection. If you are immune to any given infection, you don't need a vaccine; if you are susceptible, you may want to receive a vaccine if there is one available. This situation most commonly arises in the case of exposure to hepatitis. Many individuals have had infection without any symptoms, so the hepatitis was never recognized. But antibody tests may show that they have been infected and are immune. This spares them the need of taking the expensive series of shots.

The cells of many of the organs of the body contain enzymes or other chemicals that appear in the blood only if the cells are damaged. Damage to the lungs, heart, liver, muscles, pancreas, and prostate gland can be determined in this way. For example, enzyme tests are even more accurate than the EKG in the diagnosis of heart attacks.

If you are taking medication, it is often possible to measure the amount of it in your blood. This can be a very accurate guide to the correct dose of medication. Often the dose of medication is not critical, but certain medications used for the treatment of heart, neurologic, or psychiatric conditions require just the right blood concentration for maximum benefit and minimum toxicity. Since the necessary dose varies from patient to patient, the use of blood levels can be indispensable guides to treatment.

Body Fluids

Body fluids other than blood, those present in health or only in disease, can also be analyzed.

Urine is the body fluid most commonly examined. Among the diseases that may be detected by a urine analysis are diabetes (by the presence of sugar), infection (by the presence of pus or bacteria), and kidney disease (by the presence of protein or blood).

Spinal-fluid analysis can indicate meningitis, inflammation of the brain or spinal cord, multiple sclerosis, or a variety of other neurologic diseases. The fluid is obtained by inserting a needle between the vertebrae of the lower back. When done under appropriate circumstances, a little pain and sometimes a post-tap headache are the only complications to be expected.

Joint fluid. Arthritis sometimes causes accumulation of fluid within the affected joint. Analysis of this fluid, obtained by inserting a needle into the swollen joint, can determine, or at least suggest, the cause of the arthritis. For example, if the characteristic needlelike crystals of uric acid are seen (like a glittering spear thrown into a white blood cell), the diagnosis of gout is assured. Other crystals may also be seen. If bacteria are in the fluid, infection is present. Determination of the chemical composition of the fluid may be helpful in diagnosing other forms of arthritis.

Pleural fluid is the fluid that sometimes collects within the chest, around the lung. Heart failure, lung infections, and blood clots in the lung are some of the conditions that may cause the formation of pleural fluid. Sampling the fluid by passing a needle between the ribs into the chest can often provide clues as to the cause of the problem.

There are other body fluids that can be examined. The sperm count in semen can indicate a fertility problem; the mineral content of sweat can mean fibrocystic disease, the acid content of stomach juice can suggest or exclude the presence of peptic ulcer; the cells in abdominal fluid can show the presence of infection or cancer.

Other Body Specimens

Feces can be cultured to find infection, or examined under the microscope for the presence of worms or other parasites. In cases of chronic diarrhea, the presence of fat globules, meat fibers, or pus cells can indicate something about the nature and cause of the problem.

Kidney stones can be analyzed chemically or by X ray. Stones may be composed of calcium crystals, uric acid, oxalate, or other chemicals. The type of stone may provide a clue to the prevention of more stones.

Cells can be examined microscopically for evidence of cancer. The PAP smear of the cervix is the most common such test, but other cells can also be examined, including those found in sputum, or spinal, joint, or pleural fluids.

Cultures

If you have an infection, doing a culture—that is, isolating the infectious agent from material from your body and growing it in the laboratory—is the most accurate way to make a diagnosis. Specimens that can be used for culture include urine, blood, pus, sputum, and body fluid, or tissue obtained by biopsy.

One of the problems with cultures is that it takes time to grow the germ that is causing the infection. It takes most common bacteria twenty-four to forty-eight hours to grow numerous enough to be detectable, and it may take another twenty-four or forty-eight hours for there to be sufficient growth to allow a positive identification. But some infectious agents grow even more slowly. The bacterium that causes tuberculosis, for example, may take six weeks to become detectable.

Another problem is that some infectious agents are difficult, or even impossible, to culture; this includes some fastidious bacteria and many viruses. The diagnosis in these cases may depend on microscopic examination of biopsy specimens, or the detection of antibodies (see above).

In some cases it is possible to detect chemical components or products of the infectious agents without culturing them. Such tests may provide rapid and reasonably accurate identification of specific infections. The relatively new three-minute tests for streptococci, for example, can make a diagnosis of strep throat while you wait.

Results of cultures can be difficult to interpret. If an infectious agent is cultured from a specimen of your body that is normally sterile—such as blood, joint fluid, etc.—then that organism is surely causing your disease (provided there has been no contamination of the specimen in the collecting or transporting to the lab). But the presence of a germ in the throat, or in sputum or on the skin does not necessarily mean that it is disease producing; some bacteria just reside in these places without causing illness. The whole clinical picture must be taken into account in arriving at a diagnosis: the symptoms, the epidemiologic features, the associated findings.

A rise in antibodies to a specific infectious agent is strong evidence that an infection actually occurred. But this usually provides a retrospective diagnosis, weeks after the illness is over.

DISORDERS AND SOLUTIONS

While some repetitions may exist, in this section I have organized the discussion of tests around specific disorders. This provides an overview as well as a quick reference for specific concerns.

Heart disease. If you are suspected of having coronary artery disease— perhaps you have had some chest pain—an EKG may show evidence of a heart attack or insufficient blood supply to your heart muscle. But the resting EKG can be normal even in the presence of severe heart disease. And, of course, it may be "abnormal" even in the absence of heart disease. So you might be advised to undergo a stress test. Electrodes will be pasted on your chest so that your EKG can be monitored while you walk on a treadmill, which gradually increases in speed and slope until the exertion raises your heart rate as far as it can go (or close to that). If you have severe fatigue or chest pain or dangerous changes in blood pressure along the way, the test will be stopped. Sometimes the result of even this test is equivocal; if so, an intravenous injection of radioactive thalium can be used. The thalium quickly localizes to the heart, and appropriately done scans can show if there is impairment of blood flow to the heart muscle. If the result is still equivocal, or if you are being considered for coronary artery surgery, a coronary angiogram may be advised. This test *will* show if and how much blockage there is of your coronary arteries.

If your symptoms or a heart murmur suggest a problem with the heart valves, a chest X ray may show characteristic distortions of the cardiac silhouette. But much more detailed information can be obtained with an echocardiogram. This ultrasound picture of the heart valves and their motion may pinpoint your problem directly. If surgical repair of a defective valve is considered, or if the diagnosis is not clear, cardiac catheterization may be in order. For this test, the cardiologist passes a thin tube through the artery in your groin or arm up into the heart. By recording pressures on both sides of the valve, he can determine whether or not it is obstructed or leaking. Injecting a dye and then taking cinema X rays may show further details of valve function.

Gastrointestinal disease. As we have seen earlier, disease of the esophagus, stomach, or duodenum can often be diagnosed either by the upper GI series barium X rays or by endoscopy. The X rays are easier on you but may be less revealing than the direct view that your gastroenterologist may obtain by looking into your esophagus, stomach, and duodenum with an endoscope. Problems with your colon or rectum can also be investigated with barium X ray (barium enema) or by endoscopy.

Gallstones are most easily detected with an ultrasound examination. If that doesn't settle the issue, the next step may be to try a dye (taken by mouth) to make the gallbladder show up on X rays. Another approach is to use a radioactive tracer scan to show if the gallbladder is functioning.

Almost any gastrointestinal problem may produce a change in your stool. Traces of blood, invisible to the naked eye, can be detected chemically. Stool can be cultured for germs, examined for parasites, analyzed for fat, or examined under a microscope for evidence of pus cells or undigested meat fibers.

The liver and pancreas can be investigated by enzyme blood tests and ultrasound or CAT-scan images.

Lung disease. The chest X ray is the old reliable test. Special views and techniques can be used to enhance uncertain images, and the advent of the CAT scan adds the third dimension to the pictures.

But not all lung disease can be seen with even the best of these images. Asthma and emphysema can be more reliably detected by pulmonary function tests. The simplest and most common of these tests is spirometry. You blow as hard as you can into the spirometer, which measures the volume and force of your exhalation. Those measurements may show impairment of lung capacity or obstruction of air flow through the bronchial tubes.

Measurement of the oxygen and carbon-dioxide content of your blood indicates how effectively your lungs are functioning in their prime task of exchanging the carbon dioxide your body produces for the oxygen you inhale. This so-called blood-gas test requires sampling blood from an artery, not a vein. Usually a small needle on a syringe is used to puncture the artery in the wrist near the base of the thumb. An artery puncture is more likely to continue bleeding than a vein puncture, so the site must be compressed firmly for several minutes afterward.

If you are suspected of having a blood clot in your lung, the radioactive lung scan (with or without the use of inhalation of a trace amount of a radioactive gas) is helpful. Unfortunately there are circumstances under which the lung scan is unreliable or uninformative. Since the presence or absence of a blood clot in the lung may lead to critical treatment decisions, accuracy of diagnosis may be essential. Definitive diagnosis sometimes requires a pulmonary angiogram, an invasive and potentially dangerous test. A tube is passed through your vein into the heart and dye injected into the lung arteries, looking.for the telltale blockage due to the clot.

When there is blood in the sputum or suspicion of a tumor or other abnormality of the bronchial tubes, bronchoscopy may be the best test.

Endocrine disease. The most commonly used test for diagnosis of endocrine gland disease is measurement of the concentration in the blood of the hormones that each gland produces. These include the hormones of thyroid, pancreas, pituitary, adrenal, and parathyroid glands, and the ovaries and testicles.

A test called the radioimmunoassay combines the use of antibodies and radioactive tracers to make possible measurements of the minutest concentrations. Sometimes your doctor may administer another hormone, a chemical to stimulate or stress a particular endocrine gland to see how it responds. If a tumor of an endocrine gland is suspected, some form of imaging may be attempted. Thyroid tumors can be demonstrated by radioactive scan or by sonograms. Adrenal tumors and pituitary tumors can sometime be detected by CAT scan or MRI.

Urinary tract disease. Disease of the kidneys or any other part of the urinary tract is usually reflected in the urine. Protein in the urine may signify inflammation of the kidneys; blood may indicate tumor or stone, white blood cells may indicate infection. Culture of the urine is the most specific way of diagnosing urinary-tract infection.

IVP X rays, CAT scan, and ultrasound images may reveal distortions of size or shape of the kidneys, or the presence of tumors.

Abnormalities of the blood supply to the kidneys is revealed by angiograms, which may show cholesterol deposits or other blockage of the kidney arteries. Such blockage can sometimes cause severe high blood pressure. If discovered in time, surgical removal of the obstruction can cure these cases.

If the source of your urological trouble is the prostate gland or bladder, cystoscopy is usually the most revealing test.

Gynecologic disease. The PAP smear is probably the most commonly done test for gynecologic disorders. The scrapings from the cervix are layered on a glass slide and examined microscopically. When properly prepared and interpreted, the PAP smear can detect the earliest cell changes of cancer—when appropriate treatment results in a very high cure rate.

If there is a problem with your menstruation, the controlling hormones can be measured. The size and shape of the uterus can be determined by ultrasound. If those tests provide insufficient information, as in some cases of infertility, a hysterosalpingogram, which uses a dye that shows up on X rays and can indicate the configuration of the uterine cavity and the Fallopian tubes. Blockage of the tubes may also be demonstrated (and sometimes cured) by blowing a gas into them. The presence of ovulation can be detected by basal-body-temperature recordings.

In case of a vaginal infection, examination of the secretions may immediately show the presence of yeast, trichomonas, or other infections.

Culture of the secretions may provide more specific information, but may take days to obtain.

Sexually transmitted diseases. There are at least a dozen sexually transmitted diseases. I will refer here to tests for some of the ones most common in America. Syphilis, AIDS, and hepatitis can be detected by blood tests. In women, direct microscopic examination of vaginal secretions can diagnose trichomonas infection and can suggest chlamydia infection and the so-called nonspecific vaginitis (in which spread-by-sexual-contact is not always demonstrable). Definite diagnosis of gonorrhea or chlamydia infection requires culture of vaginal secretions or antigen tests. In men, discharge from the penis examined directly under the microscope may show gonorrhea or suggest chlamydia infection. Culture of the urethral secretions is necessary for a definite diagnosis of these infections. Pubic lice (crabs) can be diagnosed by finding the tiny creatures on the skin, or their eggs (nits) on the pubic hair. A magnifying glass or low-power microscope may be helpful.

Neuromuscular disease. Epilepsy and intermittent loss of consciousness is most often investigated by the EEG brain wave test. The information obtained from the EEG can sometimes be increased by recording it during your sleep, while you hyperventilate, or during your daily activities. Other kinds of brain dysfunction, ranging from forgetfulness to loss of mental faculties, to paralysis or coma may be investigated by CAT scans or MRI. These tests can detect strokes, hemorrhage, brain tumor, brain abscess, or generalized shrinkage of the brain. But even the best tests, unfortunately, will show no abnormality in some cases of Alzheimer's disease, brain dysfunction due to medications, accumulation of bodily toxins, hormonal or chemical imbalances, or nutritional deficiency.

Meningitis and some forms of bleeding inside the head are best diagnosed by examining the spinal fluid obtained by doing a lumbar puncture (spinal tap).

Spinal-cord problems such as tumors or the pressure of a slipped intervertebral disk can often be detected by CAT scan or the more expensive MRI.

Disease causing damage to the nerves in your body and of the muscles include Lou Gehrig's disease, diabetes, alcoholism, the toxicity of certain medications, congenital myotonia (muscle spasms), and other muscle disorders. Diagnosis is aided by appropriate blood tests, but often EMG and biopsy are required.

Modern medical tests often allow a marvelous precision of diagnosis. They also make possible detection of unsuspected disease, and they can make many treatments safer and more effective. But finding their proper use is difficult. The wrong test or too many tests may be misleading. Some tests are dangerous in the performing and others in the interpreting; virtually all are subject to misinterpretation. So understand the tests that your doctor recommends for you. Ask questions, and make sure he has good answers.

4

MEDICATIONS
Kurt Link, M.D.

Let me start by presenting an approach that may help you make good decisions about taking medications.* It is, after all, you the patient (unless you are comatose or otherwise insensible) who must make the ultimate decision about taking a prescribed medication—you who must put the tablet in your mouth, you who must swallow it. This is true whether you are the average sort of person with a modicum of skepticism and curiosity, the type who unquestioningly does as the doctor orders, or the sort that resists the introduction of any chemical into his body. Modern drug therapy offers great risks and great benefits, and your decisions will greatly influence which of these you experience.

This question of risk versus benefit is crucial to medical decision making in general and to the usage of medications in particular. You would not ordinarily consider taking a medication unless there was a potential benefit. And that potential may be great. Modern medications can influence every body function and organ. There are medications that can raise or lower blood pressure, raise or lower heart rate, raise or lower body temperature. There are medications that can put you to sleep, keep you awake, excite or calm you; there are medications that can stimulate or inhibit the stomach and intestines, the endocrine glands, the sweat glands. Some medications dilate and others constrict the bronchial tubes and the blood vessels; some medications can lower excessive blood levels of cholesterol, sugar, and uric acid. Antibiotics can kill most bacteria and some viruses; vaccines can prevent many infectious

---

*I will not discuss individual medications in this chapter except as they illustrate general concepts. There are compilations that describe specific medications in detail; these include the PDR (*Physician's Desk Reference*), the AHF (*American Hospital Formulary*), and numerous books for the layman. Also, the AMA has published patient-information fact sheets, describing commonly prescribed medications; some physicians give them to their patients along with the prescription.

diseases; diuretics can rid the body of excess fluid; analgesics can diminish pain.

But these benefits must be weighed against the risk of taking the medication. And risk there always is, no matter what the dose, no matter what the medicine. That is the essence of this chapter: how to assess the risk versus benefit of taking a prescribed medication. Some medications are, of course, intrinsically more dangerous than others as are some illnesses more serious than others. You would not want to treat a simple headache with a potentially lethal drug, but if you had an otherwise fatal disease, you might gladly take even the most dangerous medication. Some of the sorriest episodes in clinical medicine have occurred because this simple principle was ignored. Phenylbutazone (usually sold under the name Butazolidin) works like magic for the sometimes excruciating pain of bursitis. But no one ever died of bursitis. Phenylbutazone, however, can kill—on rare occasions it destroys the bone marrow and with it the patient. So I would never prescribe (and certainly never take) phenylbutazone for an affliction like bursitis. But in the past it has been commonly prescribed for just that condition. This has resulted in the rare but predictable tragic results. The antibiotic chloramphenicol has a similar devastating effect on the bone marrow in rare instances. But chloramphenicol is a potent and often life-saving antibiotic when prescribed for peritonitis and abdominal abscesses. The drug is dangerous, but for these conditions the risk is worth taking. Tragically, however, chloramphenicol was at one time widely prescribed for sore throats and even common colds, which need no antibiotic at all. And so there were needless deaths and the use of chloramphenicol was all but abandoned, even when it was needed. These are examples of the poor results that are obtained when the risk of medication exceeds the benefit. (Happily, phenylbutazone and chloramphenicol have been largely replaced by safer medications.)

THE RISKS

Let us begin this risk/benefit assessment by looking at some of the risks of taking medication. The most important of these is a potential adverse reaction to the medication itself. An adverse reaction is any undesired response. Adverse reactions may be due to allergy, idiosyncrasy, chemical toxicity, or inappropriate dosing. Some adverse reactions can be anticipated, some can be prevented, and some cannot. Any one medication may cause any or even all of these reactions.

Almost any kind of adverse reaction is commonly, but mistakenly, attributed to allergy. A true allergic reaction is due to the response of the immune defense mechanisms. In health, the immune defense mechanism fights off disease and protects you. But in an allergic reaction, this system goes haywire. It is as if all the police and firefighters were on LSD and started careening aimlessly around in emergency vehicles, smashing windows, closing down bridges, flooding the streets, creating massive traffic jams, shooting harmless citizens, and letting criminals go free.

Allergic reactions may be immediate or delayed. The immediate kind may occur if you have certain kinds of antibodies against the medication. When the antibody interacts with the medication, it sets off a chain reaction in which various cells release histamine and a host of toxic chemicals into the bloodstream. The most severe kind of immediate reaction is called anaphylaxis, a dread event that occurs within minutes and causes itching, choking, hives, collapse, unconsciousness, and death. Adrenalin (epinephrine) is the treatment for anaphylaxis. Some medications are especially likely to cause anaphylaxis—penicillin, unfortunately, among them. Anaphylaxis is more likely to occur when the medication is given by injection (especially intravenously) than when given by mouth. Don't be surprised if your doctor has little enthusiasm for penicillin shots when you have a cold.

Milder forms of immediate allergic reactions are hives, itching, cough, swelling of the tongue, swelling and inflammation at the injection site. Since the reaction is due to the presence of an antibody, anaphylaxis can only occur if you have already been exposed to the drug or some chemical component of it. Such chemicals occur in nature in the form of pollen, bacteria, and soil, so you may have been exposed without knowing it. Furthermore, modern methods of agriculture and animal husbandry involve the use of antibiotics and other chemicals and drugs, traces of which appear in the food you eat. And a trace is all it may take to sensitize you. Indeed a trace is all it may take to set off the allergic reaction. It is, in fact, characteristic of allergic reactions to be relatively independent of dose—even a very small dose can be fatal. There are exceptions: Incredibly tiny doses of some medications can sometimes be tolerated by an allergic individual. Such doses are far too small to be of therapeutic value, but they may be used to start a process of desensitization. This process is sometimes attempted if an individual is allergic to a life-saving medication for which there is no substitute.

The other form of allergic reaction is the delayed reaction. This kind occurs if certain blood cells have been sensitized to the medication. When these cells come in contact with the medication, they set up their own allergic chain reaction, which may lead to a variety of responses, including fever, swollen glands, liver inflammation, anemia, arthritis, pleurisy, and kidney malfunction. Once started, these reactions may be hard to stop and may go on for days or even weeks after the medication has been discontinued. Since the symptoms are so variable and may occur days or even weeks after exposure to the medication, these kinds of allergic reactions may be extremely difficult to diagnose correctly and may be mistaken for all kinds of other ailments. Although the delayed reactions are less dramatic than the sudden death of severe anaphylaxis, they too can be fatal. The usual treatment of delayed reactions includes the administration of cortisone or one of its chemical relatives.

The best predictor that you *will* have an allergic reaction is a personal history of previous reactions. Skin tests can also sometimes show that you are allergic. Unfortunately, neither your medical history nor any kind of test can predict with certainty that you will *not* have an allergic reaction.

Thus, allergic reactions are common and unpredictable, although the vast majority are quite mild—a transient skin rash, some itching, or a brief fever.

If you ever experience an adverse drug reaction, try to find out if it was truly an allergic reaction or not. If you have an allergic reaction to penicillin, there are large numbers of antibiotics, including some nonpenicillins, which you should avoid. This, obviously, could be a great disadvantage should you ever need such antibiotics. It would be a pity, therefore, to believe that you have an allergy when, in fact, you don't. Nausea and vomiting, diarrhea, and heartburn are common nonallergic adverse reactions. If you are allergic, make sure your medical records so indicate. Some patients even wear ID bracelets with the relevant information.

Another kind of adverse reaction is the so-called idiosyncratic reaction. This kind of reaction does not involve the immune system. Idiosyncratic reactions are unusual responses to a medication, not seen in most patients. If you have an idiosyncratic reaction, it may be due to a peculiarity in your body chemistry, such as an excess or deficiency of some chemical or enzyme. Some persons, for example, lack a protein that participates in the blood-clotting mechanism. When these individuals take the blood thinner coumarin, they develop clots and hemorrhages in the skin all over their body. Another example is those individuals who develop extreme, sometimes fatal fevers when they receive what are ordinarily harmless anesthetics. Study of these idiosyncratic reactions has, in fact, given rise to a whole discipline: pharmacogenetics. This is the study of genetic and hereditary abnormalities that cause no symptoms until the patient comes in contact with certain medications. Idiosyncratic reactions are rare. Unless there is a known family history of idiosyncratic reactions to drugs, there is no practical way to anticipate these reactions.

Chemical toxicity is another kind of adverse reaction. To some extent, almost all medications are potential poisons, and many will consistently cause unwanted toxic effects at the same time that they have their desired therapeutic effect. Aspirin regularly irritates the stomach and causes microscopic bleeding, even while it is effective in controlling fever, pain, or arthritis. Narcotics, so effective for the relief of pain, also stimulate the vomiting center of the brain. There is a very thin line between the dose of colchicine that works miracles if you have the misery of gout and the dose that will give you severe diarrhea. Some cancer chemotherapies cause hair loss or bleeding from the bladder; antihistamines cause drowsiness; some tranquilizers are addicting; some antidepressants affect the heart rhythm; some blood pressure medications cause sexual impotence. In each of these, and innumerable other cases, the medication, even when properly prescribed, will cause effects unrelated to the desired therapeutic effect. This is a property of the medication and is not an allergic or idiosyncratic reaction. This kind of toxic reaction is predictable and so should be anticipated before the first dose is taken.

Some toxicity is the result of an exaggeration of the pharmacologic or therapeutic effect of the medication. If, for example, you take enough of a medication to dry up your stomach's secretions, it will probably dry up your saliva too, causing an uncomfortable dry mouth. Or if you take an antibiotic that kills the bacteria causing your pneumonia, it may kill off the good bacteria in your intestines and vagina, causing diarrhea or a yeast infection. Blood thinners in a dose sufficient to prevent blood clots will of necessity tend to make you bleed excessively in case of an accident or surgery. In these and many other instances, the toxic effect is the same as the therapeutic effect and so cannot be prevented. But it can be anticipated and considered when decision time comes around.

Adverse medication effects may also be due to a wrong dose (from the Greek word *dosis*, meaning "gift"). Too much of a medication may be toxic; too little may be ineffective. In each case the result can be bad. I will not dwell here on the obvious errors in which the doctor writes milligrams instead of micrograms (a thousandfold difference), or the pharmacist dispenses chlorpropamide (an oral insulin) instead of chlorpromazine (a tranquilizer). But I will note that if you are in the hospital and your doctor prescribes (as commonly happens) seven different medications to be taken up to six times per day, the nurses have at least forty-two occasions daily in which they can make a dispensing error. If they are responsible for thirty patients, then it would take a miracle for everything always to go right. So the savvy patient—if he is in condition to do so—learns what medications he is supposed to take and doesn't blindly swallow a cupful of pills.

But there are more subtle dosage problems. Two people may take the same dose of medication and have very different responses. Even if an allowance is made for size (should a ninety-pound person have the same dose as a 250-pound person?) one person may be over- and another under-dosed by the comparable amount of medication. Our understanding of this puzzle is increasing, thanks to pharmacokinetics, which is the study of the movement of pharmacologic agents within, and into and out of, the body. The amount of drug that reaches its proper destination depends on a number of dynamic processes. The size of the dose that you ingest is but one facet. The amount of that dose that enters your bloodstream depends on how well your gastrointestinal tract can absorb the medication. But absorption is affected not only by how well your gastrointestinal tract is functioning, but also by the presence of other drugs or food.

It is amazing how little is known about the interaction between food and medications. What is known, however, is that most medications are absorbed better "on an empty stomach"—that is, at least an hour before, or two hours after, a meal. But if the medication is irritating to your stomach, taking it with food may be helpful. The matter is further complicated by the fact that some medications are absorbed *better* in the presence of food. These include the antifungus medication griseofulvin and some of the long-acting theophylline asthma preparations. Unfortunately there are no easy general rules to follow; one form of the antibiotic erythromycin is absorbed better in the presence of food and another is absorbed better on an empty stomach. Don't be shy about asking if food and your medication interact; but don't be surprised if your doctor doesn't know any better than you do. It may be that he is not fully informed, but often there just is nothing known about the interaction of food and specific medications.

Not all medication is taken by mouth. You may be given a prescription for a medication (usually for asthma) to be administrated via an inhaler, the correct use of which may require you to practice or get instruction. Or you may be given nitroglycerin, Cafergot, or other medication to be absorbed directly through the tissues under the tongue. This bypasses the intestinal tract and the liver, so the medication is delivered rapidly and in full strength to the tissues of the body. In recent years pharmaceutical firms have developed skin patches, known as transdermal delivery systems. These make it possible to absorb medication through the skin by putting on a Band-Aidlike patch. The advantages of this, aside from the novelty, are that sometimes a smaller dose of medication is required, the patches may last for days or even a week, and the gastrointestinal tract is not involved. Finally, there is an old but sometimes still valuable route of medication administration: the rectal suppository. If you are vomiting because of a stomach virus or a migraine headache, you may welcome the Compazine or Cafergot suppository that may give you relief.

At the same time that the medication is entering your body, your liver may be destroying it or excreting it into the bile. But instead of destroying medications, the liver sometimes converts them into drugs more potent than the original. And while that is going on, your kidneys may be filtering the medication out of the blood and into the urine at a rate that depends on how well *they* are working. These are just some of the factors, the sum total of which determine the amount of medication that is in your blood.

This situation is complicated further by the fact that certain circumstances may make you more than normally resistant, or susceptible, to a medication. For example, if your body has a lot of fat, you may be resistant to the effects of insulin. If you are depleted of potassium, ordinary doses of heart medicine like digitalis may be toxic.

Additionally, an alteration of drug receptors may alter your response to a medication. Receptors are chemicals that react with the medication; they are located in or on certain cells. This interaction between the medication and the cell's receptors is the mechanism that triggers the body's response. These receptors, if abnormal, may react excessively or insufficiently, or the receptors may be increased or reduced in number, leading to exaggerated or diminished responses. Such changes in receptors may be hereditary, or may be due to the presence of disease or the presence of other medications.

Why, you then might wonder, do not dose problems occur even more often than they do? For one thing, many of the problems noted above are rare, and most people react to most drugs in a predictable manner. For another, many medications are quite safe because the dose that is toxic is much larger than the dose that is effective, so there is room for a large margin of error. Penicillin is such a drug. Except for allergic reactions, it is such a very safe, nontoxic compound that it is common practice to administer more than may be necessary. That way you are sure to get the full benefit but still don't have to worry about toxicity.

But the key to effective dosing, especially when the dosage is critical, is close observation for efficacy and toxicity. Sometimes the action of the medication can be easily and precisely measured, as in the case of blood-thinning anticoagulants. Measuring how long it takes your blood to clot will tell exactly if you need more or less of the anticoagulant. Measuring the blood pressure will reveal the efficacy of your antihypertensive medication; measuring blood sugar indicates the adequacy of insulin dosage, etc. Similarly, when you take a drug with known toxicity—for example, one that causes a low potassium level in the blood—it may be desirable to monitor the potassium level so that this undesired effect can be detected and dealt with before it causes symptoms.

Unfortunately, the effect of a medication may not be easily measured. It may take several days of treatment with antibiotics before a serious infection can be expected to come under control. During that time, how is one to monitor the drug dose? If you are taking a medication to prevent convulsions that occur only two or three times a year, it will take that long to know if you are taking an effective dose. If your heart is very weak, it may not respond to the usual medications given in an adequate or even excessive dose. Until recently these kinds of cases were very difficult. The situation has been much improved, however, by the new technology that makes it possible to measure the amount of drug in your blood. Although not perfect, the blood level is often a very good guide to dosage. Not all drugs can be measured, and for newer drugs the ideal level has not been determined, but rapid progress is being made. So when dosing is both critical and difficult, expect your physician to check a drug blood level (and expect a big bill for this expensive test).

Another dose problem arises from the interaction of medications. When you swallow a pill, it must dissolve in your gut, be absorbed into your bloodstream, be carried by a transport chemical to its site of action, interact with the receptors of the target cells, go through your liver where it may be excreted into the bile or chemically degraded or transformed, be excreted into the urine by your kidney. Sometimes, when a medication is excreted in the bile and thus back into the intestine, it is again absorbed into the bloodstream, and goes through the whole cycle repeatedly. Many medications interact with many other medications at any one, or several, of these steps. This interaction can either exaggerate or diminish your response to one or both medications.

If you are taking multiple medications (as you would if you had, say, high blood pressure, asthma, and diabetes), the chances of an interaction occurring are great. Fortunately, most interactions are so slight that they do not affect everyday medical care, but some can be critical, so your doctor should be ever wary of possible interactions. Unfortunately slipups are easy to make and very common, so don't be afraid to raise the question: "This [new medicine] won't interact with [old medicine], will it?" If your doctor doesn't know if there is an interaction or not, he should find out.

A particularly hazardous situation arises when you are getting medication from more than one doctor. If your dermatologist, gynecologist, and internist are all prescribing for you and each doesn't know what the other is doing, watch out! Errors are also common if you have been on the same medication for a long time and suddenly need a new one for an acute condition—such as a bladder infection. Unless your doctor sits down and reviews all your medications, he may write a new prescription without thinking about a possible interaction.

A good pharmacist can be a godsend. Pharmacists are very aware of the interaction problem, and if they have your complete drug profile on hand, they can often head off trouble when you come in with a new prescription. That is one good reason to get all your medications from one pharmacy.

But perhaps the greatest dose problem comes from patient behavior. In clinical practice, the most common cause of a drug "not working" is that the patient is not taking it. This becomes a medical problem when patients—for complex reasons—say they are taking the medication when they are not. In that unfortunate situation, the physician—in his ignorance—may advise the patient to take what would really be an excessive dose, or may decide that since this drug "isn't working," he should add yet another medication.

There is a common belief that it is safer to take less than the recommended dose of a medication. This is not always true. If you take a dose too small to be therapeutic, you are exposing yourself to some hazard, no matter how small, without the possibility of benefit; the risk clearly outweighs the nonexistent benefit. Similarly, if you stop an antibiotic as soon as, for example, your throat stops hurting, the infection—not completely eradicated—may flare up again.

Instead of taking too little of a medication, you may, of course, take too much. This may come about because instructions were unclear or excessively complicated. If the directions say to take a medication four times a day, you should take four doses, spread out during your waking hours. This works for most medications. However, if it is critical that blood level of medication be strictly maintained, and if the drug does not last long in the body, the label will indicate that a dose should be taken every six hours even if it means awakening at night to do so.

If the directions say take once a day, you may not know what time of day to take the medication. I can only make mention here of some fascinating studies (of no practical importance so far) that show that the intensity of some medication effects varies with the time of day that the medication is taken. But if no specific information is available, use common sense. If drowsiness is a side effect, taking the medication at night may be helpful. If the medication makes you urinate often, however, taking it at bedtime may interfere with your sleep. If you miss a dose, you may not know whether to forget it or double up. This will vary from medication to medication. If the medication is long-acting, doubling up will usually be desirable, but if it is short-acting, doubling up may cause toxicity. But there may be exceptions, and you will have to check with your pharmacist or physician to be sure. In any case, once you decide when to take your once-a-day dose, it is good to take it at about the same time every day.

You may be tempted *deliberately* to take a larger-than-recommended dose in an attempt to achieve a result not provided by the smaller dose. Or there may be a partial response that you seek to intensify with extra medication. The idea "If a little medication is good, more medication is better" can be an even worse idea than "Less is safer." The benefit obtainable from any medication is limited, and is often maximal at or near the recommended dose. Increasing the dose may produce toxicity without further benefit.

THE BENEFITS

The benefit of taking a medication will depend in part on the purpose for which it is taken. A medication may be prescribed for a variety of reasons: to cure, to replace a deficiency, to control or arrest the progress of disease, to relieve symptoms, to prevent illness. Or a medication may be used as a placebo. Or finally medication may be taken for its own sake. Although these categories sometimes overlap and are not all-inclusive, we can use them to help structure this presentation.

Cure, of course, is the ideal achievement. You take your medicine, your illness is cured, and you are as good as new.

Does this ever occur? Sometimes. The example that comes closest to this ideal is probably the use of antibiotics to cure an infection. Gonorrhea, pneumococcal pneumonia, staph blood poisoning, kidney infections, all may be cured by the right antibiotic. Actually the antibiotic does not entirely cure you; it reduces the number of bacteria to the point that your own body defenses can destroy the remaining invaders. Some cancers, including some leukemias and some forms of Hodgkins disease, can be completely eradicated; patients are truly cured. Duodenal ulcers tend to heal themselves, but when they don't, antacids or drugs that inhibit acid secretion may lead to healing, as does the use of Sucralfate that protects the stomach lining. In each case, the ulcer heals, and in that sense you are cured (until and unless the ulcer recurs). If you have a problem with infertility, and medication induces ovulation and subsequent pregnancy, you have been cured of your infertility.

But just because you get better while taking a medication does not, of course, mean that it is the medication that cured you. If you have an ailment from which you will get better by yourself, any medication that you take, even if it is totally inert, may create the illusion of cure. There are many cures of this type, including cures for the common cold, back sprains, intestinal upsets, headaches, fatigue, and minor emotional problems.

A true cure is the exceptional, but ideal, result. If you are taking a medication in the hope of affecting a cure, you are reaching for the ultimate benefit, and you have good reason indeed for taking the medication (unless the ailment is trivial and the medication potentially lethal—but more of that later).

Taking a medication to correct certain deficiencies sometimes comes very close to being as good as cure. I have seen more than one individual with a thyroid hormone deficiency slowly transformed from being thick-tongued, coarse-featured, and slow-moving to bright, busy, and cheery. As long as that individual continues to take the thyroid medication, he will be perfectly well, but as soon as he stops, he will slowly slip back into his previous morbid state.

Vitamin B_{12} monthly shots will keep at bay indefinitely the devastating symptoms of pernicious anemia, which is caused by the body's inability to absorb B_{12} from food. Replacing thyroid and B_{12} gives near perfect results, in part because the body requires a more or less constant supply, which can be provided by oral medication (such as thyroid) or injection (B_{12}). The replacement of some other deficiencies provides a far less perfect result because the body requires an ever-changing amount of the needed substance, and this need cannot be met by any existing medication delivery system. For example, some patients with diabetes lack insulin, but treatment leaves much to be desired because no reasonable number of injections can mimic the natural ebb and flow of insulin secretion. To some extent the same is true for the treatment of the cortisone deficiency caused by the absence of the adrenal gland (Addison's disease). There are, in the natural state, hourly variations in the blood cortisol level as well as variations induced by stress of any kind. This effect cannot be duplicated by any dose of pills. But even in these cases, the replacement, however imperfect, can sustain a life that would otherwise quickly end.

For anyone with a deficiency disease, medication is a must.

Medicines may also be taken to arrest or slow the progress of an ailment that cannot be cured. The treatment of hypertension is a good example. Untreated, hypertension may cause symptoms such as headache and nose bleeds, but more importantly, it sometimes leads to strokes, heart attacks, and gangrene. Cure of hypertension is the goal, but in over 90 percent of cases, the cause is unknown and so is the cure. But there are medications that can lower blood pressure and prevent these complications. As long as you take your medication, your blood pressure stays down, but as soon as you stop, it will usually go back up. The medication does not cure, but it halts or slows progression of the disease.

Other examples include rheumatoid arthritis which, in its progressive form, can be slowed by treatment with gold and certain other medications. The destructive effect on the eye of the elevated ocular pressure of glaucoma can be slowed or prevented by eyedrops or oral medication. Other examples include the treatment of diabetes, chronic kidney failure, some cases of kidney stones, some blood disorders, epilepsy, and others.

Some of the medications used to slow progression of disease have considerable toxic potential, but the benefit of preventing strokes or maintaining joint function may justify considerable risk taking.

Let us now consider taking medication solely for the relief of symptoms. In this case the medication does not cure and does not in any way affect the progress of the disease. Medication taken for the relief of pain is usually in this category. Most sprains, minor fractures, headaches, back pains, menstrual cramps, and other common painful conditions will generally clear up just as fast if you take medication or not. Literally tons of medication are consumed daily for purely symptomatic relief, including headache powders, all the cold remedies and cough syrups, most allergy remedies, most sleeping pills and tranquilizers, medications for diarrhea, nausea, or abdominal cramps.

How great a risk should you take for the relief of symptoms? This will depend on the severity of the symptoms and the riskiness of the medication. If you have a mild headache, taking a couple of aspirins seems quite reasonable. But if you have an ulcer that flares up if you take aspirin, you might conclude that it is better to put up with the symptoms than to take the medicine. If you are passing a kidney stone, however, you will not think along those lines; you will reach for *any* pain relief no matter how toxic. In the case of a heart attack or a potentially lethal injury the pain may in itself worsen the condition; relief of pain may actually be life saving. But these are the exceptions.

Insomnia or chronic nervousness and anxiety can cast a pall over your life and dampen all your pleasures. The temptation to take medication for relief from these symptoms may, therefore, be great. But the benefits, which are often less than hoped for, must be weighed against the risk of habituation and chemical dependency. This problem presents one of the most difficult medication decisions, and may require the most careful consideration. If you are the patient, your judgment may be blunted by the intensity of your distress. Unfortunately, physicians also sometimes have trouble in this area. Some are so afraid of inducing a drug-dependency problem that they resist use of these medications beyond reason. Others dispense them willy-nilly just to get a troublesome patient out of their hair. A good decision may be hard to make. As always, the risk must be measured against the benefit.

Another reason to take medication is for the prevention of disease. The benefit in this case must include both the likelihood of contracting the disease and its severity. The use of rabies vaccine is a good example. Rabies is a fatal disease, so any potential exposure must be taken seriously. Until a few years ago, however, the vaccine was derived from animal sources and so caused some very severe allergic reactions. If you were bitten, you tried to assess the risk of getting rabies. If you were bitten by a bat, for example, you might ask, How many cases of rabies from bats have occurred in *this* county in the past ten years? Or, has anyone *ever* gotten rabies from a pinpoint-sized bat bite on the tip of the left thumb? If the risk seemed minimal, you might conclude that it would be safer not to take the vaccine. But now there is a much safer vaccine derived from human cells; it is expensive, it is not altogether painless, but it is safe. Now, *any* risk of rabies probably warrants prophylaxis.

Smallpox prophylaxis presents a contrasting case. When smallpox was prevalent, no one in his right mind would refuse the protection of the vaccine. True, there were rare serious reactions to the vaccine, but smallpox is frequently lethal and the risk of getting smallpox was great. However, as the number of cases of smallpox diminished (thanks to the vaccine), the risk of getting smallpox got ever smaller. But the risk of reactions to the vaccine was constant. A time came when the risk/benefit ratio tilted in favor of no vaccine; indeed in this country vaccination is no longer recommended. Smallpox has since been totally eradicated (the most glorious story of modern medicine), so the smallpox vaccine question is moot.

Similar but less striking changes in the risk/benefit ratio of other vaccines are taking place, including such common vaccines as measles, polio, and diphtheria. In each case, the vaccine is so effective in preventing the disease that the relative risk of the vaccine is increased. This has led to increasing concern by some parents about the vaccination of their children, even with the common DPT (diphtheria, pertussis, tetanus). Some serious reactions to these vaccines have occurred. This had given rise to so much litigation that several pharmaceutical houses had stopped vaccine production three years ago and a potentially dangerous shortage of vaccine ensued. The specter of a return of some old epidemics was abolished only by some protective legislation and some changes in manufacturing and selling practices.

So far we have been discussing only vaccines as our example of taking medication to prevent disease. Vaccines are perhaps the purest example of this use, but there are many other medications taken to prevent disease.

If you are going to travel to a place where malaria is common, you will be advised to take some prophylactic medication. The medication recommended will depend on which type of malaria is present. In 1985, if you had made plans to go to certain parts of Africa that have a relatively resistant form of malaria, you would have been advised to take Fansidar. But serious adverse reactions to Fansidar have occurred, bringing the risk/benefit ratio close to 1—that is, the risk and benefit appear to be almost equal, by most calculations. So now you would probably be advised to obtain Fansidar—but not to take it. Unless, that is, you think you might be experiencing the very first signs of malaria. At that point your risk of getting malaria has risen (you might, in fact, already have it). So now the risk/benefit ratio has changed again; you must take the medication.

Birth-control pills are another medication taken for the prevention of disease. This may not be the way most people view birth-control pills, but to the physician or epidemiologist, pregnancy can be viewed as if it were a disease—that is, an undesired result. The benefit, of course, is not getting pregnant. The value of that benefit depends on several factors. If getting pregnant means you are going to have an abortion, then the pill will protect you from the risk of abortion. If you intend to carry the baby to term, then the hazards of pregnancy and delivery have to be taken into account. These in turn will depend in part on your age, health, income, marital status, and past obstetric history. Other benefits include no fear of pregnancy, possibly better sex, and a reduction in certain infections and female cancers.

The likelihood of your getting pregnant without the pills must also enter into the calculation. If, for any reason, your risk of getting pregnant is very small, the potential benefit of the pill is accordingly reduced. Furthermore, since there are other ways to avoid becoming pregnant, the risk/benefit ratio of other contraceptive methods must be considered.

What are the risks of the pill? The known risks are spelled out in the product brochures—high blood pressure, diabetes, blood clots, heart attacks, liver tumors, and a host of chemical changes of no known consequences. The risk rises significantly with increasing age, especially if you also smoke and already have a predisposition to one of the adverse effects of the pill.

Analysis of the risk/benefit ratio is obviously a complex business here. If you are young, have no predisposing illnesses, and do not smoke, if you are unable or unwilling to use barrier methods such as condoms and diaphragms, the pill is clearly for you. If you smoke, are approaching forty, and have a tendency to high blood pressure, the pill is clearly not for you. Often, of course, the issue is not so clear-cut; you may have to confer with your physician at some length and ponder the question before coming up with the right answer for you.

Now consider medication as placebo (Latin: "I shall please"). The placebo, in its pure form, is a pharmacologically inert material given to the patient in the guise of an effective medication. In the old days physicians commonly gave patients "sugar pills" to please them, or to satisfy their desire for treatment even if none was available or none was needed. Such overt duplicity is not acceptable today, and the placebo is rarely used in this form. More likely, your doctor will give you a prescription for a medication, even if it is unlikely to have a significant pharmacologic effect. He may prescribe vitamins or a tiny dose of sedative or B_{12} shots. In each of these cases he more or less consciously relies on the placebo effect to please you. If he actually believes in the pharmacologic value of the medication, the placebo effect will be intensified, because the power of the placebo comes from the strength of the belief in it.

If you believe in the healing properties of the placebo, it may indeed heal you, and if you fear it, it may indeed harm you. Many studies have demonstrated this strange business.

The placebo can make you feel better or worse; it can make you vigorous or lethargic; it can cause nausea, headache, and vomiting; it can cause hives; it can lower your blood pressure, your blood sugar, your cholesterol; it can affect the rhythm of your heart and the rhythm of your breathing. Because of the placebo effect 30 percent of patients enthusiastically prescribed an absolutely worthless new treatment will improve, regardless of the condition being treated. The improvement may be very incomplete and will be transient, but it will occur, and it will be real. This is why many new treatments initially hailed as "breakthroughs" quickly become discarded; the placebo effect wears off, and their real value, or lack thereof, becomes manifest.

Even though you might not ordinarily knowingly take a placebo, we can still try to analyze the risk/benefit ratio. The benefit is some relief of symptoms. What about risk? At first thought, one might be tempted to consider an inert drug risk-free; this would make *any* benefit of a placebo attractive. But a placebo is not risk free. To begin with, various side effects can occur, as we have already noted. Furthermore, if you are given a placebo and respond well to it, the search for the cause of your ailment may be prematurely ended, and some important condition left undiscovered. The eventual failure of the placebo will tend to undermine the relationship with your doctor, even if you don't discover that you were given a placebo. If you do make this discovery, the relationship may be destroyed. Furthermore, if we recognize that in the long run, the placebo has no real benefit, then the risk/benefit assessment clearly comes out negative.

It might be argued that some situations do justify the use of the placebo. Why not reach for whatever little relief a placebo might provide for the hopelessly or terminally ill individual to whom there is nothing better to offer? My personal answer is that there is something better to provide than deception; hope and comfort can take forms other than a capsule or injection.

So, if you are like me, you do not want your doctor to prescribe a placebo. But *every* prescription has a placebo effect, and your physician would be remiss to be unaware of it or to ignore it. He can and should try to use the placebo effect to reinforce the pharmacologic effect. A medication provided in a half-hearted way with unclear instructions and uncertain benefits may not work as well as the same medication presented in a positive, reasonably optimistic light. But that is different from prescribing a placebo as placebo. Don't encourage your doctor to use a placebo: If you insist on getting a prescription when he doesn't think one will be helpful, he will be tempted to please you. Let him know that you want medication only if it is clearly beneficial, and let him know you want to know how the medicine is supposed to work.

A final note. Knowing about the placebo effect does not at all negate it. Some people are placebo responders, and some aren't. I am a responder. As soon as I swallow a pill, I feel somewhat different, even though I know that the medication hasn't even begun to enter my bloodstream. So if you feel stronger after taking the vitamins or B_{12} shots, or if you sleep better after taking some herbs from China, it could be a pharmacologic effect—or it could be the placebo effect.

Now we come to a medication problem even more difficult than the placebo: the use of medication for its own sake. Ordinarily, medication is taken to achieve certain ends, such as cure of disease, etc. But on occasion this goal becomes eclipsed by a need to take the medication for pleasure, comfort, or relief that is unrelated to the original therapeutic intent. The most typical example is the habituation or addiction to pain-relieving medicine. Perhaps you were taking medication for the relief of some painful condition. Perhaps in time the condition is cured. Your need for the medication ended; there was no longer any reason that you should want to take the medication. And yet you found that you craved it. Or you may have taken a benzodiazepam tranquilizer (of which Valium is but one of many) for relief of anxiety. With the passage of time you may have found that the anxiety was still or again there, or not there—it didn't matter. You begin to take the medication for its own sake, the original anxiety being no longer relevant. Painkillers and tranquilizers are not the only medications that can be craved for their own sake. Sleeping pills, diet pills, stimulants, antihistamines, and some hormones can fall into this category.

You may not realize that you are beginning to take medication for its own sake as you gradually drift from medical need to medication need. If your doctor begins resisting your requests for the medication, if you continue to take the medication even though it is not helping, if you continue to take the medication even though the original problem has been resolved, if you continue to take the medication against your doctor's orders—you may have passed from therapeutic use to dependency. The medication has become the problem instead of the solution.

A closely related problem is the use of medication in an attempt to obtain relief even when the medication is not working and continued usage may be harmful. If you have fallen into this unhappy situation, your behavior may resemble that of the individual who has developed medication dependency. You take the medication against orders; you are secretive about how much you take; you attempt to get more by going to multiple sources; you are oblivious to the potential harm the medication may do.

Asthmatic patients have died because they used their inhalers excessively even when the relief obtained was very brief and was followed by increasingly severe symptoms; patients with rhinitis may get caught up in a cycle of increasing rebound nasal congestion after taking ever larger or more frequent doses of decongestants until they have near total nasal obstruction; patients with arthritis may not be able to quit taking their cortisone even though the side effects become more severe and dangerous than the arthritis ever was. Laxatives, diuretics, and even some blood-pressure medicines are among the other medications that may give rise to this problem. Again, the medication has become the problem instead of the solution.

If you find yourself taking medication for its own sake, recognize that you are in a dangerous circumstances and get help. If your physician can't help you—or, worse, if he is a contributor to the problem—ask for a consultation or seek a second opinion on your own. These medication problems can be difficult to solve, and the sooner you get help, the better.

COMMONLY USED MEDICATIONS

Having discussed some generalities about the use of medication, let us now take a brief look at some of the major classes of commonly used medications. The selection is certainly not complete, but comprehensive references (some of which are mentioned in the beginning of this chapter) are available. In this discussion I use the generic or chemical name for medications when that is commonly known or when there are multiple brand names for the same medication. It would be too cumbersome to list all five or more trade names for one medication. But where the medication is only available as one or two brand names, and has an unfamiliar generic name, I use the brand name. Brand names are capitalized, generic names are not.

Antibiotics

These are the drugs that kill bacteria and some other organisms that cause infections. The original antibiotics of the 1940s, such as penicillin and streptomycin, were substances manufactured by living organisms (such as yeast and fungi), which killed other organisms—mainly bacteria. But the term "antibiotic" is now used for almost any anti-infective medication, including the sulfa compounds and drugs partially or wholly synthesized in the laboratory. There are now over fifty antibiotics available, and their number seems to grow daily. Correctly choosing and using antibiotics has thus become so difficult that it sometimes takes an infectious-disease specialist to make the right decision.

Viruses, unfortunately, remain largely untouched by antibiotics. The few exceptions include AZT (originally named azidothymidine, then zidovudine; the trade name is Retrovir—the AIDS virus is a *retrovirus*), which is partially active against the AIDS virus, and acyclovir, which is active against the herpes virus. Many studies have shown that doctors often prescribe antibiotics for patients with common colds and other viral infections, even though antibiotics don't help. If this happens to you, you are being needlessly exposed to the risk of an adverse reaction. Also a problem is the growth of bacteria that are resistant to antibiotics.

The ideal situation occurs when your doctor knows what organism has infected you and so can prescribe an antibiotic that is known to be effective against it. If, as is likely, more than one antibiotic is effective, then the safest, and—all other things being equal—the cheapest should be chosen.

Cardiovascular Drugs
High blood pressure. The blood pressure is the sum of multiple dynamic forces, which include the forcefulness of the heart's pumping action, the total volume of blood in the body, and the degree of spasm or relaxation of arteries and veins. Each of these factors is partly under the control of the brain, nerves, hormones, and kidneys. The medications used for treating high blood pressure act on one or more of these factors; often a combination of more than one medication will provide the best response. The major classes of antihypertensive drugs are the diuretics (to control blood volume and also relax arteries), the beta blockers (which decrease the force of the cardiac pump), the drugs that affect the brain's influence on the nervous and endocrine systems, the calcium channel blockers and vasodilators (which relax the arteries), and the ACE inhibitors (which favorably affect the concentration of blood-pressure-raising hormones).

Each class and each drug has its individual merits. Each class and each drug also has its individual side effects. The side effects of these medications include fatigue, low potassium, sexual dysfunction, depression, drowsiness, gout, diabetes, fluid retention, dehydration, arthritis, excess hair growth, and swelling of lips and tongue.

The goal of treatment for high blood pressure, then, is to find the medication or combination of medications that provides maximum blood pressure control with minimum side effects.

Heart disease. Coronary artery disease is America's most common heart ailment. Angina, the pain associated with narrowed coronary arteries, can sometimes be controlled with medications such as nitroglycerin, the beta blockers, or the calcium channel blockers. Each, in a different way, decreases the heart's need for oxygen and/or increases the supply.

Coronary artery disease and other forms of heart disease may damage the heart muscle sufficiently to cause the heart to fail as an effective pump. Some drugs make it easier for the heart to pump the blood by relaxing the arteries and so lowering the resistance that the pump has to overcome. These are the vasodilator drugs. Others help the heart by decreasing the volume of fluid that the heart has to move—these are diuretics. And some medications, like digitalis and its derivatives, strengthen the heart muscle itself.

A whole other class of drugs known as antiarrhythmic drugs are useful in correcting abnormal heart rhythms, some of which are potentially lethal. It has recently been found, however, that some of these drugs actually create or worsen the abnormal rhythm that they are supposed to prevent or treat. This has greatly complicated their use, and hospitalization is sometimes necessary to use these medications safely.

Gastrointestinal Drugs

Acid. Many stomach conditions are caused by or exacerbated by stomach acid. These conditions include ulcers, esophagitis, and heartburn. There are three kinds of medications used to combat stomach acid. Antacids such as Maalox and many others neutralize the acid. Other medications decrease the formation of acid. Zantac and Tagamet are relatively new and very powerful drugs of this class. A third class of medication, which includes Carafate, coats the stomach lining and protects it from the effects of the acid.

Motility disorders. Diarrhea, constipation, and abdominal cramps may all be symptoms of abnormal contraction of the intestine—the motility disorders, so named because there is disruption of the normal sequential contractions that propel the bowel contents along. A variety of antispasmodic drugs, as well as high-fiber bulking agents such as Metamucil, may be helpful. Many laxatives work by decreasing the intestines' ability to absorb water. They thus cure the constipation by adding additional dysfunction to the already present motility disorder. They may also be habit forming. That is why fiber (dietary or supplement) is the preferred treatment.

Neurologic Drugs

Antiepileptic drugs. Phenytoin (diphenylhydantoin, Dilantin) and phenobarbital have a long history in the treatment of the ancient malady, epilepsy. These drugs are still among the most effective medications available, although newer agents are sometimes better. The availability of drug blood levels has made the use of new and old agents safer and more effective. The old practice of using multiple drugs has given way to the ideal of monotherapy, in which the physician attempts to find the single most effective drug and to prescribe it in the most effective way so that no other medication is required.

Migraine. There are many medications used to relieve the migraine sufferer. Based in part on the unproved theory that migraine headaches are caused by abnormal constriction and relaxation of the blood vessels in the brain, many migraine remedies contain derivatives of ergotamine, a powerful blood vessel constrictor. This is often combined with pain killers and caffeine (for no known reason). Another approach is to try to prevent the headaches. Calcium channel blockers (diltiazem, verapamil, nifedipine, and others) and beta blockers (including propranolol and many others) will not help if you already have a migraine headache, but they may prevent them if taken regularly.

Vertigo, vomiting. Vertigo, the whirling around kind of dizziness, and many cases of nausea and vomiting are caused by disturbances in the brain or inner ear. Antihistamines and some medications in the tranquilizer category may be helpful.

Psychoactive Drugs

Antipsychotic drugs. Also known as major tranquilizers, these are the medications that have allowed severely ill persons formerly confined to straitjackets and the locked wards of the old state psychiatric hospitals to live halfway normal or comfortable lives. They may also be of great benefit to less severely ill patients who nonetheless have psychotic symptoms. They are also useful in some acute delirious states due to toxic brain disturbances. Most of these drugs are phenothiazines, but there are several other groups also. All these drugs are potentially toxic, causing cardiac, liver, and neurologic problems, but in appropriate cases, this is a risk well worth taking.

Minor tranquilizers. These drugs are both so useful and so troublesome. Most are in the benzodiazepam class (Valium and many others), and these are all associated with habituation and abuse. Most physicians feel that they do have a place in the short-term treatment of anxiety. Their role in more chronic states is controversial. Buspar, a relatively new minor tranquilizer, is said not to cause dependence, but it can cause other psychological side effects.

Antidepressants. The antidepressant drugs are one of the greatest gifts of modern pharmacology. The sicker the patient, the more dramatic the response. Imipramine (Tofranil), one of the earliest and still one of the best of these drugs, has been followed by a host of others in the search for a medication with faster onset of action and less toxicity. Some progress has been made but most often the toxicity is changed rather than diminished, and a great potential for suicide is still a problem with many of these medications.

The depression associated with manic-depressive illness seems quite different from the more usual depressive illness. Patients with this illness sometimes get worse with conventional antidepressants but do very well with lithium. The antidepressants are also very helpful in some patients with disabling phobias.

Sedatives. Sleeping pills. A difficult subject, because insomnia is a difficult problem. All sedatives tend to be habit-forming, and all sedatives lose their efficacy with continued use. Insomnia is often classified as transient, short-term, or long-term. Transient insomnia lasts for two or three days and usually requires no treatment. Short-term insomnia, usually caused by temporary stress, can be treated with a short-acting sedative but should not be continued for more than three weeks. Long-term insomnia requires a complete diagnostic evaluation, as it may have many causes. Sedatives are rarely helpful.

Painkillers

If you are in severe acute pain caused by perhaps an injury, childbirth, kidney stone, or heart attack, adequate doses of narcotics almost always will be helpful. But large problems arise when the painful condition is chronic, as in chronic headaches, low back pain, or arthritis, or the condition is recurrent, as in menstrual cramps or migraine. The narcotics and their derivatives all have addicting potential and tend to lose efficacy with repeated or continued use—that is, tolerance develops. In chronic cases, therefore, nonpharmacologic methods of pain control are often better than narcotics.

For less severe pain, aspirin, acetaminophen (Tylenol), and a whole new group of nonsteroidal anti-inflammatory (NSAIDS) drugs provide a nonaddicting welcome relief. They have their own side effects, of course, mainly stomach and kidney problems. There are about a dozen of these drugs, including ibuprofen (Motrin, Advil, Medipren, Rufen), Indocin, Clinoril, Tolectin, and Anaprox.

Respiratory

Coughs and colds. When, as is the case for colds and coughs, there are a large number of medications for a given condition or symptom, it means either that none of them work very well or (less often) all work equally well. Cough medicines usually contain codeine, which is, of course a controlled (narcotic) drug or dextromethorphan, which can be bought without prescription. Since coughing helps clear the bronchial tubes, it should at times not be entirely suppressed.

Cough medicines often also contain antihistamines and decongestants to help with sneezing, running nose, and stopped-up ears. The relief these medications provide may be partly undone by the drowsiness, nervousness, or nausea that they sometimes cause. In any case, if the symptoms are due to a cold, they go away in a few days.

More difficult is the treatment of cold-type symptoms due to allergy. These symptoms do not go away in a few days, and the side effects of the usual medications can be a real problem when taken for weeks at a time. Nasal sprays containing cortisone derivatives or cromolyn may be helpful. Desensitization with allergy shots is another approach.

Asthma, emphysema, chronic bronchitis. Theophylline preparations (aminophylline, Theo-Dur, Slo-bid, and many others) strengthen the diaphragm and dilate the bronchial tubes by causing chemical changes within the cells. The beta agonist (ephedrine [not much used anymore], terbutaline, albuterol, and others) also dilate the bronchial tubes (by stimulating nerve endings) and work well with the theophyllines. The beta agonists can be given in tablet form or preferably by inhalation. If these treatments are insufficient, cortisone preparations can be used. Oral or intravenous cortisone preparations are most effective but may cause severe side effects if taken continuously or repeatedly. Cortisone derivatives taken by inhalation are somewhat less effective but much safer. Other medications used for asthma include the inhaled Atrovent which helps to dilate the bronchial tubes in yet a third way, and cromolyn which interrupts the allergic response which is often a component of the asthma attack.

Endocrine

Hormones may be used to treat deficiency, or may be used as pharmacologic agents—that is, in doses larger than normally present in the body.

All the classic endocrine glands, including the thyroid, pituitary, adrenal, ovaries and testes, and the insulin-producing islet cells of the pancreas, may become diseased to the point that they stop producing sufficient hormone. This deficiency can be corrected by administering the hormone by injection or by mouth. The goal is to supply the hormone in a way that mimics the natural state. To the extent that the goal is met, the patient is restored to full health. In the case of thyroid deficiency, it is easy to come close to success. But, as we noted in the discussion of medication as replacement therapy, the results of replacing deficient adrenal cortex hormones and insulin are far from perfect.

Hormones may also be used as pharmacologic agents. Birth-control pills are used to treat unwanted fertility; other hormones or hormone simulators are used to treat unwanted infertility; cortisone and its derivatives are used to treat immune disorders, allergic disorders, and arthritis; estrogen may be used to slow the growth of prostate cancer and testosterone may slow the growth of breast cancer. In each of these cases the patient receives more than the natural amount of hormone. It thus has dangers and side effects just like any other medication.

I should note here that the old endocrine story, so tidy, of the pituitary master gland controlling the six or so other discrete endocrine glands, turns out to be a great oversimplification. The interactions among the glands is complex, and endocrine "glands" are turning up all over the place, and the number of known hormones seems to increase daily. There are hormone-producing cells in the gastrointestinal tract, in the lung, in the brain, and in other places that they are not supposed to belong. The same hormone pops up in different places, accomplishing different things. The questions far outnumber the answers, but the near future will undoubtedly bring new therapeutic uses for some newly discovered hormones.

Metabolism

Many bodily ailments are caused at least indirectly by an abnormal accumulation or deficiency of some bodily chemical. In many cases this can be corrected by appropriate medication. These medications affect the body's metabolism—that is the absorption, formation, destruction, or excretion of that chemical.

Uric acid. When abnormal amounts of uric acid accumulate in your body, you are prone to kidney stones and gout. A number of medications, of which probenecid is one, cause the kidney to speed up the excretion of uric acid and so restore balance toward normal. If your kidneys are not working well or if you have been forming kidney stones, such medication may not work or may worsen the problem. In that case, allopurinol can be used; it prevents the formation of uric acid and restores balance in that way.

Cholesterol. By now every one knows that high levels of cholesterol predispose one to heart disease and hardening of the arteries. Some drugs prevent the absorption of cholesterol—these are the resins—and they are moderately effective but require large multiple doses of bad-tasting expensive medicine. Cholestyramine is the most commonly used. Nicotinic acid, probucol, and others lower the cholesterol level by different mechanisms. A new agent, lovastatin, interferes with the body's manufacture of cholesterol and is very potent in lowering blood cholesterol. It is assumed, but not yet proved, that it, like cholestyramine, will decrease the heart attack rate.

Sugar. High blood sugar is, of course, the cardinal manifestation of diabetes, and insulin is the cornerstone medication for its treatment. But insulin can be given only by injection because it is broken down in the intestine, and even if it weren't, it could not be absorbed because it is such a large molecule. There are, however, several medications in pill form which can lower blood sugar in some cases, if the pancreatic islet cells are still capable of producing some insulin. These so-called oral insulins are not at all like insulin. They work in part by stimulating the body to increase its own insulin production and in part by making body tissues more sensitive to insulin.

Minerals. As in the case of hormones, these agents can be used to treat deficiency states, or can be used as pharmacologic medications.

Iron deficiency, probably the most common mineral deficiency, causes anemia (and other less clinically apparent effects). Treatment with oral iron is safe and effective, although sometimes it causes some gastrointestinal discomfort. Iron is highly toxic if taken in excess and is one of the most common and serious causes of poisoning in children. Childproof caps and storage of iron pills out of reach of children are important preventive measures. Sodium deficiency can be replaced, depending on the circumstances, with salt pills, table salt, or intravenously. Potassium deficiency, often caused by diuretic "fluid pills," can be replaced from food sources or medication, most often in the form of potassium chloride pills, tablets, or liquid. Calcium deficiency occurs usually after menopause or as a complication of treatment with cortisone. It most often shows itself in the thinning and fragility of the bones that occurs in osteoporosis. Unlike the other minerals we have discussed, in which the deficiency can be measured as a low level of the mineral in the blood, in the case of osteoporosis the blood level of calcium is normal, but the amount of calcium in the bones is decreased. Oddly enough, once the calcium is lost from the bones, it cannot be replaced simply by giving calcium. Success of calcium therapy, therefore, depends on providing plenty of calcium years before the osteoporosis starts. Other mineral deficiencies are rare and occur in the setting of unusual circumstances such as prolonged malnutrition or as a result of some modern medical therapies like use of the artificial kidney or prolonged life support with intravenous nourishments.

Minerals are sometimes used as pharmacologic agents to treat illness. Everyone agrees that fluoride prevents cavities (although some would argue that this is replacing a deficiency, not treating an illness). Lithium is effective in some psychiatric disorders. Magnesium, which has largely been replaced by newer drugs, is still a good sedative and antihypertensive medication, especially in alcoholic delirium and, oddly enough, eclampsia of pregnancy. Zinc has been reported to be good for treating colds, but this has not been widely accepted and its potential toxicity is unknown.

It should be noted that many minerals have a lethal toxic potential and so must always be administered with great care. In some disease states, minerals, including iron, lead, and calcium, accumulate to toxic levels; sometimes these excesses can be treated with a variety of medications.

Vitamins. Vitamin deficiency causes a host of troubles, including disease of skin, brain, nerves, heart, bone, and virtually every organ and tissue. When disease is caused by a vitamin deficiency, treatment (with a few exceptions) is safe and sure. Clinically evident deficiencies are most often the result of malnutrition, but may be due to medical treatments, or diseases that interfere with absorption of the vitamin (as seen in pernicious anemia and some diseases of the intestine) or the metabolism of the vitamin (as seen in advanced kidney failure).

Vitamins are sometimes used as pharmacologic agents. A few examples include vitamin C, which has been used to prevent colds, vitamin D to treat osteoporosis, vitamin E to treat hardening of the arteries, and vitamin B_6 to treat carpal tunnel syndrome (pain or tingling in the hand). The value—or lack thereof—of many of the pharmacologic uses of vitamins are obscured by hot controversy, egotistical rhetoric, self-serving personal and financial interests, and, above all, lack of good data. (See Chapter 7, Nutrition, for further discussion.)

Immunizations

There are two types of immunization, active and passive. Active immunization is the stimulation of the immune system to produce antibodies

Medications

against a given infectious agent. Passive immunization is the administration of preformed antibodies.

Active immunization. Active immunization is achieved by administration of a vaccine that stimulates certain cells to produce antibodies, which will prevent infection. Since this process takes days or weeks, there may be considerable delay between vaccination and protection from infection. Because of this, active immunization is good for prevention of disease, but often ineffective in treatment of disease. The immunity induced by active immunization, once it occurs, tends to be long-lasting.

Active immunization may be induced by live vaccines or nonlive vaccines. Live vaccines consist of living organisms that are a relatively harmless variant of a disease-causing germ. Administration of a live vaccine causes an infection that stimulates the body to produce antibodies, which are directed against both the vaccine organism and the disease-producing one. An unusual feature of some live vaccines is that the infection can spread. Oral polio vaccine virus, for example, can spread from the vaccinated individual to other household members. Such spread will immunize other susceptible individuals. But spread of smallpox vaccination to household members with eczema or rashes can cause a very severe illness, about as bad as smallpox itself. The chief advantage of live vaccines is that immunity tends to be long-lasting—often a lifetime. The disadvantage of live vaccines is that they do produce an illness, albeit a very mild one that often goes entirely unnoticed. But if the immune system of the vaccinated person is impaired, the mild illness may be anything but mild. Because of this, patients with AIDS or certain cancers, and those receiving some cancer chemotherapy, should not receive live vaccines.

Commonly used live vaccines include smallpox (now obsolete), oral polio (there is also a killed polio vaccine), rubella (German measles), measles, and mumps.

Nonlive vaccines consist of killed whole organisms or a chemical extracted from them. Many commonly used vaccines are of this type, including influenza, hepatitis, rabies, and pneumococcal pneumonia. Although these vaccines are perhaps somewhat safer than live vaccines, they tend to be a bit less effective. The antibody responses may not be as intense, and immunity may decrease after a number of years, making booster shots necessary to maintain immunity.

The vaccines against diphtheria and tetanus are called toxoids because the vaccine is derived from the poisonous toxins that these bacteria produce. The antibodies that the toxoids induce neutralize the toxin but do not directly attack the bacteria.

Passive immunization. Active immunization stimulates the body to produce antibodies; passive immunization is accomplished by injection of preformed antibodies. In the old days these preparations were derived from immunized animals and were dangerous to use, but now much safer preparations, derived from human sources, are available. These antibody preparations, called immune globulins, are extracted from the serum of actively immunized donors. There are commercially available immune globulins directed against numerous infections, including hepatitis A, hepatitis B, tetanus, and rabies.

Unlike active immunization induced by vaccines, passive immunization provides immediate protection, but the protection lasts only as long the antibodies last, which is a matter of days or at most weeks. Sometimes the appropriate vaccine and immune globulin are administered together so that by the time the immune globulin wears off, the vaccine has begun to work.

THE COST FACTOR AND THE USE OF GENERICS

We now come to the cost of medications and the use of generics. Before 1938 you could buy any medicine you had the money to pay for, except for narcotics. But in 1938 the Food and Drug Administration (FDA) created a distinction between drugs available only by prescription and those available over the counter (OTC). Although this had been the aim of the FDA for some time, it was the Elixir Sulfanilamide episode of 1937 that created the climate that made passage of those regulations possible. The Massengill Company, a long-established drug house, marketed the established sulfa drug, sulfanilamide, in a new, liquid form. The solvent vehicle, diethylene glycol, was quickly found to be lethal. The first six gallons of this new medicine killed over a hundred people. Before a year had gone by, the FDA ruled that certain drugs could be dispensed only if prescribed by a physician, although this ruling would not have prevented the Elixir Sulfanilamide disaster. The intent was, of course, to protect the public from toxic drugs. The effect was that consumers were no longer considered competent to select their own medicines (1). Drug manufacturers would decide which medications could be sold only by prescription, and doctors would decide which consumers would get prescriptions. This ruling caused much confusion: The same drug could be classified as a prescription drug by one manufacturer and as an over-the-counter drug by another. There was also persisting concern about efficacy, toxicity, and purity of medications. These issues were addressed by the 1951 Durham-Humphrey amendment to the Federal Food, Drug, and Cosmetic Act. It was now the government that would determine which drugs could be sold only by prescription and which over the counter. Thanks to this legislation, the consumer is barred from direct purchase of almost all new medications and indeed most old ones too.

Since most drugs can be obtained only by a doctor's prescription, doctors have become the main conduit of brand-drug sales, which are now over $1 billion annually. Physicians have also become the main target of the industry's intense and sophisticated advertising. To the extent that they are successful in persuading doctors to prescribe their products, the pharmaceutical firms determine which medication you buy. And they try very hard. Besides being exposed to the usual professional journal advertising, every doctor gets free cassette tapes, video tapes, news magazines, and medical journals. A $100 honorarium for spending a couple of hours in a "marketing seminar" (with a buffet of course) is not unusual, and sometimes there is even a weekend at a resort to help a pharmaceutical firm develop new ways to market its products. There are also rosters of paid speakers, some quite expert in their fields, who will give lectures to the hospital staff and sometimes at special dinner meetings at the finer restaurants in town. And then there are the "representatives." No more the day of the detail man, who marched into the doctor's office with a memorized sales pitch and a supply of samples. Now there are bright, good-looking men and women with backgrounds in pharmacy, psychology, or nursing. They know their product in depth and tactfully teach the doctor about the new medication and how to prescribe it. Unchanged is the practice of leaving samples. The doctor's sample closet, if he has one, is regularly stocked with literally hundreds of dollars worth of medication. Samples sell; the pharmaceutical firms know this. And the drugs they sell, of course, are the ones most profitable. It is the new drug, the "breakthrough," that gets most of the attention. Retrovir (for AIDS) costs about $1,000 per month; some of the newer antibiotics cost several hundred dollars per day; Activase (for dissolving heart attack-producing blood clots) costs almost $1,000 per dose. These are the drugs that are under patent and so can be legally sold only by the patent holder or with the patent holder's blessing. The patent lasts for seventeen years (not renewable) from the date of synthesis, but it may take a decade or more before a new drug wins FDA approval for marketing. Because this may shorten the period of effective patent rights, the 1984 Drug Price Competition and Patent Term Restoration Act was written to include a provision that guarantees at least five years of market exclusivity after FDA approval (2). During this period the patent holder has a monopoly on the medication and will try to maximize profits, recoup the development and research costs, and try to equate, in the doctor's mind, the brand name with the medication itself.

When the patent does run out, other firms can start to manufacture and sell the medication, using their own trade name or the generic name. Newer drugs commonly have three names: chemical, generic, and brand names. A commonly used antihypertensive, for example, has the chemical name 1-(Isopropylamino)-3-(1-napthyloxy)-2-propanalol hydrochloride; the generic name propanalol; and the brand name Inderal. The chemical name tells those knowledgeable about such things the chemical structure of the drug. The generic name, somewhat less technical, is also assigned to the chemical entity. The generic name is not a brand name or trade name, and it is not the property of any company. Before 1962 the firm that originated a drug could assign the generic name, but since then a unique generic name has been assigned to each drug entity by the United States Adopted Name Council composed of physicians, pharmacists, and drug manufacturers (2). The generic name usually suggests something about the chemical composition of the drug.

The patented drug is referred to as the standard or innovator drug; the same medicine sold by other makers after the patent expires is called a generic drug or generic. These generics are often priced *by their manufacturers* far below the original patented brand-name drugs.

During the 1940s and into the 1950s, generics were widely dispensed in lieu of the brand-name drugs, often without the prescribing physician's knowledge. In the 1950s more than forty states enacted antisubstitution laws or regulations which forbade the substitution of generics for brand-name medications.

The innovator drug manufacturers undoubtedly played a major role in passage of the antisubstitution acts. They were, of course, driven by their own economic interests, but they were able to bolster their self-serving arguments by demonstrating that generics sometimes differed significantly from the brand-name drug.

Tablets, capsules, and liquid preparations of the same medication may have different effects. Even tablets manufactured by different methods may have different effects. A typical sugar-coated tablet contains only 8.3 percent active ingredients. The remainder consists of binders, excipients (fillers), lubricants, and coatings (4), all of which can affect the rate at which the tablet dissolves, how well it is absorbed, and the intensity of its effect. Tablets made by different manufacturers may differ significantly in all these respects, but as long as all of the products have the same weight of active medication, they are said to be *generically* equivalent. By demonstrating that serious therapeutic differences exist between some generics and the brand-name drug, and by accusing smaller generic houses of producing inferior, substandard medications, it was possible to induce the legislators to pass antisubstitution laws and regulations.

Although the facts did not change, the political climate did. In the 1970s there were intense pressures by government, health insurers, and consumer advocates to control the cost of medical care. Substitution of generics for brand-name drugs was seen as an attractive step in this direction. The result of these pressures was the repeal of the antisubstitution statutes and their replacement with regulations that encouraged the use of generics. In many states, for example, the pharmacist may at his discretion substitute a generic unless the physician specifies that he wants only the brand named to be dispensed. In some states he must certify that it is medically necessary to dispense only the brand-name medication.

The same old objections to substitution were once again raised, of course. (An analysis of the scientific, social, and political forces involved in this long struggle is described in a wonderful paper by Neil J. Facchinetti [3].) But the 1984 Drug Price Competition and Patent Term Restoration Act defined new procedures to expedite marketing of generics and set up new standards for generics. These standards include testing new generics in human volunteers and comparing blood levels of the generic to the blood levels achieved with the standard brand-name drug. Critics say these standards are too loose. The volunteer tests, for example, use as few as eighteen subjects, who are between ages twenty-one and thirty-five, are healthy, within 10 percent of ideal weight, and in the fasting state. One standard, the so-called 75–75 rule, requires that 75 percent of the test results be no more than 12 percent and no less than 75 percent of the result obtained with the brand-name drug. Other standards allow specific variance between generic and brand-name drugs. For some medications (warfarin) a 10 percent variance is allowed; for others (antipsychotic drugs) a 30 percent variance is allowed (5).

What is one to make of all this? Although no clinically significant problem with any generic meeting these new standards has been uncovered, the standards do in fact allow considerable variation between generic and brand-name drugs. Problems may yet come to light.

There are other potential problems with generic substitutions. Each manufacturer's tablet may have a different appearance and a different name. Different drug stores may dispense different brands of the medication and sometimes the same drugstore may switch from one generic brand to another. This can cause confusion for both patient and physician. A prescription written for Bactrim DS may ultimately become a bottle bearing the label Biocraft TMX; the subsequent telephone exchanges among patient, physician, and pharmacist may resemble a conversation among the Three Stooges.

In their attempt to fight off the generics, the innovator drug houses rely on advertising and some tricks of the trade. One of these is to come up with novel, sometimes patentable, new delivery systems. If the standard tablet is being marketed generically, they may come up with a long-acting formulation that is not available generically. Or with a transdermal skin-patch delivery system. Or with a microburst capsule that releases its content one tiny pellet at a time. Some of these products have real advantages; others are as necessary as curb feelers on a DeSoto.

In my opinion generics as now approved by the FDA are generally acceptable. Extra caution may be appropriate, however, for those medications that are potentially life-saving, and those that have a small difference between therapeutic and toxic doses. Among such medicines are anticonvulsants, many cardiac drugs, some hormones, and antidepressants. You want exactly the same effect every time you get your prescription filled; you might, therefore, want to get exactly the same product every time. In any case, you ought to weigh carefully the theoretical risk of therapeutic variance against the benefit of less cost.

And now we come to one of the most peculiar aspects of this whole subject: the retail cost of medication.

To have any hope of success, the manufacturer of generics must be able to sell the medication for substantially less than the brand-name manufacturer. Usually this is no difficult task, since, as we noted, the brand-name drug cost is set to maximize profits as long as its manufacturer holds a monopoly. It is not uncommon for the brand-name manufacturer to lower prices when the patent expires and the generic competition sets in, but generics, on the whole, are still much cheaper. This ought to mean, one would think, that you can get your generic prescription filled for less. That, after all, is the avowed purpose of all the statutes and regulations that encourage generic substitutions. But it turns out that at the retail level, when you pay the pharmacist, generics are sometimes only very little less expensive (6) and at times are even more expensive than the brand-name drugs (7).

Prices vary greatly from one pharmacy to another, and one pharmacy may be cheaper for some items but more expensive for others. Some observers frankly blame this on unfair practices by pharmacists (6), (8), but the pharmacists hotly deny these allegations (9), (10). Whatever the merits of the various arguments, it is demonstrably true that although on the whole generics are cheaper, having a generic prescription in hand does not guarantee the large savings that you might expect. To maximize savings, you need to shop around, perhaps by telephone, and find where you can get the best buy on each medication. You might even want to consider mail-order pharmacies for medications that you will need a lot of; major savings are sometimes possible. This kind of aggressive shopping does have its own cost, of course, in time and effort spent, and does require you to forgo the sometimes important benefit of having a personal pharmacist who is familiar with all your medications.

5

SURGERY
Kurt Link, MD

HISTORY OF SURGERY

The Neolithic fossil evidence is clear. Stone Age man practiced surgery. There is no written record, of course, to tell why Neolithic man (or woman?) chiseled those holes in the skulls of his fellows. But he did, using a stone ground sharp or a splinter of obsidian. Trephined skulls have been found on various continents, and the partial regrowth of the missing bone shows that some of the patients survived. The "surgeon's" motive might have been to let out demons, or to fulfill some other religious ritual, but it was, in crude form, the same operation performed today by neurosurgeons in cases of head injury.

The first *written* record concerning the practice of surgery is found in that 4,000-year-old Babylonian document known to all high school students—the Code of Hammurabi. Surgeons were having troubles even then. If his patient dies, the Code calls for the amputation of the surgeon's hand—although there is no apparent documentation that this penalty was actually exacted; indeed this provision could not have been much enforced or there would have been no surgery.

Even then, social issues were entangled in medical practice and education. The penalties of the code applied only if the patient who died was a free man. In the case of a surgical death of a slave, the surgeon had only to recompense the owner for the value of the slave. In ancient Persia, at about the same time, a surgeon had to operate successfully on three infidels before he was allowed to practice. If he failed the test, he could never again practice surgery.

With the rise of the ancient Greek civilization, there was a concentration and development of medical knowledge. The earliest mentioned healer was Aesculapius or Asclepius, who was probably a mortal physician who later became deified. His followers were mystic healers with a remarkable record for cures, in large part because they never took on desperately ill patients. The patients were healed by magic and mysticism in Asclepian temples. From this cult a sound theory of medicine gradually grew, and the mystics in time became physicians/priests. Indeed, Hippocrates, the great practitioner who was born and worked on the Greek island of Cos, was a physician of the Asclepian school. His oath, now 2,000 years old, is known to all. He was physician, surgeon, and pharmacist. He left seventy volumes of his writings, some dealing with surgery, setting fractures, and bandaging wounds. He separated science from religion; this was probably his greatest contribution to civilization. He wrote that the art of medicine has to do with "the disease, the patient, and the physician." The gods were not included. The Asclepian physician/priests had become physicians.

In the second century A.D. Claudius Galenus, known as Galen and as Paradoxopoeus—the Wonder Worker—taught that there is a teleologic explanation for every phenomenon. He was a brilliant, charismatic physician, unequaled in his time. But he was also very dogmatic. He espoused and elaborated the ancient Greek humoral theory of disease. And, although he dissected animals, he never studied human anatomy and, indeed, opposed the dissection of human flesh. His influence lasted for 1,500 years and tragically stifled the growth of knowledge and especially the study of anatomy, and hence surgery.

With the fall of the Roman Empire in the fifth century, Europe entered the Dark Ages. For a thousand years, disease was once again seen as the work of demons and the devil and as the wages of sin. The plagues swept back and forth across the continents leaving mountains of putrid corpses heaped in the city streets. Fearful and helpless, the survivors cried out to God and flagellated themselves in hopes of salvation.

Surgery was considered dirty and lowly work, and was left to barber surgeons, who carried their crude and filthy instruments from town to town, performing blood lettings, tooth extractions, and removal of bladder stones (in those days a very common and painful affliction). To the summons of clashing symbols crowds gathered on the village green as the barber surgeon prepared to operate. The spectacle and screams of the patients had the same fascination then that an auto accident has today. As soon as the work was done, the barber surgeon hastily departed, to leave the patient/victim to recover on his own or have complications and die.

The late Middle Ages saw the beginnings of Europe's great universities. It was the Age of Scholasticism. Medical, philosophical, and all other issues were decided by intellectual and theoretical inquiries.

Surgery

But in 1543 the intellectual ground began to shift. Andreas Vesalius published *De Humani Corporis Fabrica*, the first complete textbook of anatomy and arguably the most significant text in all medical history. It was based on his own observations and study of human anatomy. Anatomy was no light undertaking; Vesalius had to exhume corpses, perform secret midnight dissections, and defy the law, the wisdom of the ancients, and even, many would have said, the will of God. He had the courage to trust his own observations and the artistry to make those observations believable. He was the father of modern anatomy.

Within thirty years the father of modern surgery, Ambroise Paré, began to publish his observations, clearly recording them and making a rational change in the practice of surgery. At the age of twenty-six, this is what he did at the siege of Vilaine in 1536.

> I was at that time a freshwater surgeon since I had not yet seen treated wounds made by firearms. It is true I had read in Jean deVigo's first books of *WOUNDS IN GENERAL*, chap 8, that wounds made by firearms are poisoned because of the powder. For their cure he advised their cauterization with oil of elders mixed with a little theriac. To not fail, this oil must be applied boiling, even though this would cause the wounded extreme pain. I wished to know first how to apply it, how the other surgeons did their first dressing—which was to apply the oil as boiling as possible. So it took heart to do as they did. Finally, my oil was exhausted and I was forced instead to apply a digestive made of egg yolk, rose oil, and turpentine. That night I could not sleep easily, thinking that by failure of cauterizing, I would find the wounded in whom I had failed to apply the oil, dead of poisoning. This made me get up early in the morning to visit them. There, beyond my hope, I found those on whom I had used the digestive medication feeling little pain in their wounds, without inflammation and swelling, having rested well through the night. The others, on whom I had used the oil I found feverish, with great pain, swelling and inflammation of their wounds. Then I resolved never again to so cruelly burn those wounded by gunshot.

What is so remarkable about this account? Consider that it was written 453 years ago. The "scientific method" was an idea more than three hundred years into the future. Superstition was the order of the day. The concept of infection, or microorganisms did not exist. And yet here was young Pare, already a compassionate man, open minded, and using his own observations to guide his therapy.

Paré also learned, and taught, how to ligate blood vessels, thus controlling bleeding and allowing soldiers to survive amputation. This was one of the turning points in the history of medicine that pointed to the advent of modern surgery. Paré's contributions were not limited to the battlefield and operating theater. One of his major achievements was to translate Vesalius' great work from Latin into the vernacular (French) and so make it available to all surgeons.

But Paré was the exception, and barber surgeons continued to practice their trade until the eighteenth century. During that 200 year span the Age of the Scientific Revolution saw Harvey's discovery of the circulation, Van Leeuwenhoek's microscope, the beginnings of embryology and biochemistry. In England the surgeons and barbers developed separate guilds, and in 1800 the Royal College of Surgeons was established. But even today the surgeon is "Mister," not "Doctor," and even today the jokes harken back to ancient days: "The surgeon knows nothing but does everything; the physician knows everything and does nothing."

As the nineteenth century dawned, much was known about anatomy, physiology, the classification and natural history of disease. But surgery was a bloody, brutal business hastily conducted under the stress produced by the agonized patient's screams, and usually resulted in immediate death due to shock and hemorrhage or delayed death due to infection.

The era of modern surgery could not begin until three great barriers fell—infection, pain, and shock due to loss of blood. Modern surgery had to wait for antisepsis, anesthesia, and blood transfusion.

Pasteur did not discover microbes and bacteria (leading to the later formulation of the germ theory of disease) until the latter half of the nineteenth century, but astute observers recognized that the surgeons themselves were somehow transmitting puerperal fever, blood poisoning, and gangrene. Holmes and Semmelweis were two such observers.

In 1842 Oliver Wendell Holmes published his paper, *On the Contagiousness of Puerperal Fever*. He recognized that the surgeon's dirty hands were transmitting infection from one patient to another. Even though the article was published in *The New England Journal of Medicine*, his work was ignored by the whole profession except for the obstetricians, whose leading lights and spokesmen denounced his work.

At almost the same time, a Hungarian obstetrician at the First Obstetrical Clinic at Vienna Hospital, Ignaz Philipp Semmelweis, noticed that the postpartum ward attended by the students who came directly from the cadaver dissections had a much higher rate of puerperal fever than did the ward attended by the midwives. Later a close friend of his died after nicking himself with a dissecting knife—of an illness that had many of the features of puerperal fever. Semmelweis then understood that the cadavers were the source of infection, which was being carried on the hands of the students, and he required them to wash their hands before attending the patients. So great was the resistance to this idea that he literally had to block the entrance to the ward and force the students to wash their hands in the basin of chlorine that he held. The death rate on that pestilential obstetric ward fell from 12 percent to 3 percent. But he was seen as an obsessive zealot who disrupted the routine of the clinic, and he was not very diplomatic in his attempts to persuade. His appointment at the clinic was not renewed, and he had to return to Budapest.

In the 1860s, Joseph Lister, in Scotland, made observations similar to those of Semmelweis. But by this time Pasteur had discovered the microbe, and so observation was reinforced by theory. Lister found that wounds treated with carbolic acid, which killed bacteria, healed without infection. In 1867 he presented his paper, *On the Antiseptic Principle in the Practice of Surgery*, to the British Medical Association meeting in Dublin. The clinical use of antiseptic technique had arrived. But widespread acceptance was delayed by some bizarre detours. Lister, like most innovators, was an intense man. He began by soaking instruments in carbolic acid and washing the patient's skin with it before and after surgery. His method, as he finally developed it, required a steam-powered motor to spray a fine mist of carbolic acid throughout the operating room, and so the surgery was carried out in an atmosphere of fumes that caused cough and headache for all in attendance. So intense, and at times excessive, was the ritual that many soon lost sight of the rationale. Surgeons began to use carbolic acid as if it were magic, because they did not understand the germ theory of disease. They would douse a wound with carbolic acid and then stuff it with a filthy dressing. When infection set in, they denounced "Listerism" as a failure and a hoax. This retarded but did not stop the general acceptance of antiseptic methods.

Listerism was practiced until the last decade of the nineteenth century. At about that time, antisepsis (something that combats infection) was replaced by asepsis (entire absence of infection). Instruments were sterilized by steam, floors and walls cleaned, sterilized garments were worn, and finally, in 1890, William Halsted introduced sterile gloves. The carbolic acid ritual was replaced by the glove, gown, and mask ritual. The second major barrier to modern surgery had fallen.

Earlier, at the time of Holmes' and Semmelweis' observation about the spread of infection, the first barrier—the intolerable pain of surgery—had also fallen. But once again, the discovery had to be made repeatedly, and resistance had to be overcome before the truth could be seen and widely accepted.

In the early 1800s nitrous oxide (laughing gas), now widely used by dentists, was a popular recreational drug at carnivals and on college campuses. The users often amused onlookers by their hilarious antics.

In 1844, in Hartford a dentist, Horace Wells, was attending a sold-out public demonstration of the wonders of laughing gas. His companion, a volunteer performer, struck his shin a sharp blow while under the influence, but felt no pain. Wells was able to grasp the significance of this observation and persuaded a surgeon to allow him to demonstrate a tooth extraction at the Massachusetts General Hospital. But the volunteer was an obese man who was resistant to nitrous oxide, and the demonstration ended in a humiliating failure complete with laughter and catcalls.

Wells's former associate, William T. G. Morton, was shortly afterward introduced by his chemist to a different gas, ether. Morton tried it, with results so dramatic that he was later allowed yet another demonstration at the Massachusetts General Hospital, and that did it. "Gentlemen, this is no humbug," said the awed surgeon, Dr. John C. Warren. Never mind the subsequent bitter, vicious, and petty feuding and lawsuits (never settled because of the onset of the Civil War) about who was the true discoverer. On October 16, 1846, anesthesia was born.

But in part because Dr. Morton kept the nature of his ether a secret (disguising it with perfumes), the Medical Society, in an extraordinary meeting, prohibited its further use. Finally Morton revealed his secret. Some saw Morton as a great benefactor of mankind—indeed the French Academy of Science so designated him on a specially made gold medal. Others saw him as a mercenary character who attempted to use his stolen discovery for his own benefit. In any case, legend has it that Morton fell so low that he tried to pawn his gold medal before he died in poverty and obscurity, in 1868. Thus did the pain barrier to surgery fall.

Treatises on the history of blood transfusion commonly cite the ancient rituals that indicate a belief in the power of blood. The ancient Egyptians bathed in blood for strength and rejuvenation, and it is said that Roman spectators rushed to drink the blood of the fallen gladiators. Some authorities state that the first blood transfusion occurred in 1492 when Pope Innocent VIII, on his death bed, was given the blood of three young boys. The record is unclear, but it is probable that the Pope drank the blood and did not receive a bona-fide transfusion. In any case, the boys died, the Pope died, and the doctor was disgraced.

The first real transfusion was described by Andreas Labavius in 1615. He wrote:

> Let there be present a robust healthy youth full of lively blood. Let there come one exhausted in strength, weak, enervated, scarcely breathing. Let the master of the art have little tubes that can be adapted one to the other; then let him open an artery of the healthy

one, insert the tube and secure it. Next let him incise the artery of the patient and put it into the feminine tube. Now let him adapt the two tubes to each other and the arterial blood of the healthy one, warm and full of spirit will leap into the sick one, and immediately will bring him to the fountain of life, and will drive away all languor.

The date of this record suggests that, incredibly, Libavius made his discovery before William Harvey described the circulation of blood—one of the great milestones of medical history. In 1628 Harvey published *Exercitatio De Motu Cordis,* which was an account of his proof that the blood does circulate, that its movement is purely mechanical, produced by the heart, which functions as a pump. That discovery led to further experimentation with blood transfusion. In 1667 Richard Lower transfused a healthy but mildly insane man with the blood of a lamb. It appears that this was a demonstration before the Royal Society and was more of a show than a therapeutic procedure. The recipient of the blood was paid 20 shillings to allow the transfusion. The demonstration, although before a distinguished group of scientists, caused some merriment. One observer wrote that "It gave rise to many pretty wishes as of the blood of a Quaker to be let into an archbishop and such like."

Not long after that Jean Baptiste Denys of Montpellier, Louis XIV's physician, transfused a boy sick with fever with lamb's blood. He appeared to improve, and transfusions soon became fairly common. Using the blood of an animal was the dominant idea of the time. It was believed that characteristics of the animal would be engrafted on the human recipient. For this reason, the supposed calming effect of lamb's blood was favored. On the other hand there was fear that horns or other animal characteristics might appear. Insanity, lung and bowel afflictions, and the debilitation of old age were considered indications for transfusion. A novel idea was the settling of marital discord by reciprocal transfusion of husband and wife.

We now know that animal blood is always incompatible with human blood, and that such transfusions could not possibly have been helpful. Recipients of animal blood probably survived, when they did, because the amount transfused was so small. Disasters were common, and when Denys' fourth patient died, Denys was tried for murder. He was acquitted, but transfusions were outlawed, and it was a hundred years before they were tried again.

In 1829, the English obstetrician James Blundell saved at least four women from death due to postpartum hemorrhage by transfusing them with human blood. He used a syringe to draw blood from the donor and inject it into the recipient. But success was a hit-and-miss affair. If the blood happened to be compatible, the patient benefited; if not, there were reactions, often severe and deadly. This remained true for the rest of the nineteenth century, and blood was used only as a last desperate measure to save the life of a bleeding patient. Transfusion of animal blood also continued.

At the turn of the century, the Nobel-prize winning work of Karl Landsteiner catapulted blood transfusion into the modern era. He discovered that the blood of one human may be incompatible with that of another. He simply took blood samples from himself and five of his staff members, and separated the red blood cells from the serum. He then tried mixing the cells and serum in various combinations. In some cases the red cells formed a solid, nonfluid clump, and in other cases the cells remained in an even suspension. It quickly became apparent that there were three main blood types, now known as A, B and O. Mixing like types caused no clumping and no reaction; mixing unlike types sometimes caused clumping and transfusion reactions. In one stroke, the science of blood transfusion was born. It was forty years before the Rh factor was discovered (also by Landsteiner). Today there are fourteen major blood group systems known, and the ABO and RH incompatibility are the most important causes of transfusion reactions. Problems remained, but these were solved in relatively short order. The clotting of blood during the transfusion was a major practical problem until the anticoagulant citrate was discovered. Fevers were frequent until it was found that they were often due to bacterial contamination, which could be prevented by careful technique. Charles Drew's discovery of plasma, which could often be used instead of whole blood, is credited with saving tens of thousands of lives in World War II. Finally the techniques of blood storage allowed the development of the modern blood bank, which made it possible to have blood always available.

Thus, thanks to the efforts of people of widely differing backgrounds—rural Georgia, Vienna, Paris—the era of modern surgery began, along with its subsequent refinements and advances, some of which will be described below.

RISK–BENEFIT RATIO

Every year 15 million Americans (one in fifteen) have some kind of surgery. In virtually all cases the patient gives consent to the surgery, often formally and in writing. In recent years, thanks largely to malpractice suits, surgeons have been paying much more attention to obtaining consent, because failure to obtain consent can be grounds for malpractice suits if the surgery does not go well. And consent, to stand up in court, must be *informed* consent, and not just a hurried signature at the bottom of an uninformative, incomprehensible, or unread document. Regrettably, to "cover" themselves,

Surgery

the doctors and hospital administrators have transformed these consent forms into long frightening lists of every conceivable dread complication. If you were to believe that the complications listed are likely to happen, you would never have surgery, just as you would never take so much as an aspirin if you read about all the potential and rare toxic effects.

If you are contemplating surgery, consent forms of this type do not help you decide what to do. The real decision making goes on informally, in discussion with your surgeon, primary care doctor, friends or relatives. My purpose here is to help you make your decisions as rational and as informed as possible. Unfortunately, as we shall see, the necessary data for entirely rational decision making is often unavailable and even unobtainable, so every decision is made with some uncertainty.

Central to rational decision making, in all areas of medical practice, is a consideration of risk and gain, or the risk–benefit ratio of any course of action (or inaction). So, one question to ask is, "What is the risk of surgery?" The question, in isolation, is meaningless. Is a 0.5 percent mortality rate low enough, is a 10 percent mortality rate too high? The answer depends entirely on the benefit. If the alternative to surgery is almost certain death, as for example if you had profuse internal hemorrhage due to an injured spleen associated with other major injuries, a 10 percent mortality rate would be acceptable: The risk of dying during surgery is 10 percent, but it is much less than the risk of no surgery. The benefit is a 90 percent greater likelihood of survival.

But consider another example. Suppose you have heartburn, and are plagued by bitter-tasting acid and little bits of food regurgitating into your mouth after meals, but have experienced no dangerous complications. Suppose further that you are told that a surgical procedure could repair your hiatus hernia and so eliminate your symptoms. Would a 0.5 percent mortality rate for such surgery be acceptable, or might even that be too high in this case? If you consider only life and death, surgery loses. There is a 0.5 percent risk of death due to surgery but no benefit in terms of survival since, in this case, the condition itself carries no risk of death.

Life and death, of course, are *not* the only considerations. The benefit/risk analysis must also take into account the quality of life before the after surgery, and must reflect your values. In the case of the hiatus hernia example, is the pleasure, now lost, that you used to get from a good meal so great that a 0.5 percent chance of dying is well worth taking? Would you prefer to suffer along with the pain in your arthritic hip or undergo major hip surgery with its attendant pain and hazard? Would you rather live for six months, at home, your body intact, or live for eighteen months after major, noncurative surgery predictably requiring extensive hospitalization, treatments, and tubes in your body? The answer to these kinds of questions will greatly affect how you weigh the balance between risk and benefit. The answers cannot come from statistics or doctors—they come only from you.

So far we have considered surgery versus no surgery. But you must also ask, "What are the alternatives to surgical treatment?" It may be possible for you to be treated by radiation, diet, chemotherapy, or medications. In that case rational decision making will require you to compare the risk and benefits of surgical versus nonsurgical treatment. In the arthritis of the hip case, for example, medication may greatly diminish the pain, but all medications that are effective in arthritis have dangers of their own, including internal bleeding, kidney problems, and others. So the dangers of surgery must be weighed against the dangers of the medication, and the benefit of surgery (ideally, a pain free new hip) compared to the benefit of medication (a significant relief of pain). Similarly, in the case of the hiatus hernia, symptoms may be controllable by nonsurgical means. If you put blocks under the head of your bed, take antacids often, and take medication to suppress acid production by your stomach, the symptoms may subside. Which is better: surgery with its risk, or a life of pill taking with its cost, inconvenience, and possibility of side effects?

Comparing surgery to nonsurgical treatment can, paradoxically, be made even more difficult by medical progress. Consider coronary artery bypass graft (CABG). When the coronary arteries are partly blocked by cholesterol deposits, chest pain known as angina may develop. In the old days (ten to twenty years ago) the only available treatment was the administration of medications, which were often not effective. With the advent of CABG surgery, it was found that bypassing the blocked area with a portion of one of the dispensable veins in the leg would almost always stop the angina. So far, so good. It was easy to tell that the operation worked. Before the operation, the pain was severe with the slightest exertion; after the operation the patient could once again take out the garbage.

Then came the question: "But does the operation prolong life?" This was not so easy to tell. Suppose, without surgery, the average life expectancy is five years and that with surgery it is eight years. It will take at least eight years to find that out, and then only if a large number of patients are available for observation. Several years ago just such studies were completed—in the United States and in Europe. In all cases it was found that with certain severe, critical blockages of the coronary arteries, patients who had bypass surgery lived longer than those treated with medication alone. But during the study years and since, look what happened.

Several new drugs appeared, which are much more powerful and effective than the older ones, thus improving the results with medication alone. At the same time, however, advances were made in surgical techniques, including use of an inflatable balloon that stretches open the arteries without requiring surgery in the usual sense at all. So the question you ask today, when contemplating bypass surgery, is not the one that was answered just a few years ago. Now you want to know, which is better, balloon angioplasty or use of the newer drugs? The study to answer that question has not been done, and probably never will because therapy is simply changing too fast.

Recognizing, then, that an informed appraisal of risks and benefits has its limitations, let us nonetheless review some of the known risks and benefits of ordinary modern surgery.

RISKS

Surgical risk appraisal is a very uncertain science. In many cases data and statistics are available that will very accurately predict the outcome for certain surgical procedures for a group of patients, but are not very useful for predicting the outcome for an individual. Lumping all United States surgeries together, the risk of death is about 1 percent to 2 percent (1). A hernia repair in an otherwise healthy adult under age fifty carries a mortality rate that is less than 0.1 percent, or less than one death in 1,000 operations. But death for the unlucky individual represents a mortality rate of 100 percent. Nonetheless, available statistics provide a starting point in assessing risk.

In the case of a high risk situation, the surgeon commonly calls upon a medical physician and anesthesiologist to help estimate risk and, more importantly, minimize it. Some risk factors such as high blood pressure or severe anemia can be eliminated or modified before surgery. Other risk factors, such as a recent heart attack, can alert the physicians to likely complications that can be prevented or at least detected early. So considering risk may help decide whether or not to have surgery.

The risks associated with anesthesia and surgery may be divided into patient-related risks and provider-related risks. Let us consider these in turn.

Patient related risks.

Each patient has a unique combination of attributes that affect his surgical risk. These attributes include gender, the condition for which surgery is proposed, age, unrelated coexisting ailments, medication history, and nutritional state.

Gender is a factor. Men have a higher surgical mortality rate than women. This may be because men have a higher likelihood of heart disease and are more likely to be cigarette smokers with all that implies; men may also delay seeing a doctor and thus have more advanced disease.

The condition for which surgery is required will obviously affect mortality. A hernia repair is less risky than a gallbladder removal, which is much less risky than repair of a ruptured aorta.

Age, one would intuitively suspect, is also a risk factor. And indeed, patients over age seventy have a ten times higher surgical mortality than do young adults. But the excess deaths appear to be due to the presence of coexisting disease, especially heart disease, and senility, or other severe mental impairment. If such factors are excluded, it is very hard to demonstrate that age in and of itself affects mortality. Indeed, heart surgery and other major operations are commonly successful in the otherwise healthy patient even into the eighth and ninth decades of life.

The presence of coexisting ailments is a major risk factor. Chief among these is heart disease. If you have surgery within three months of having had a heart attack, you have a 30 percent chance of dying or having another heart attack. If you can postpone surgery for six months after a heart attack, the rate of dying or a second heart attack associated with surgery falls to 5 percent (2).

If you have high blood pressure, you are also at greater risk, especially if the pressure is not well controlled. If you are contemplating surgery, make sure that your blood pressure is under good control well before the date of surgery. Make sure that you have explicit instructions about how long you should continue to take your medication. Usually it should be taken right up to the time of surgery, but check with the prescribing physician.

Lung problems may increase surgical risk and definitely increase the likelihood of postoperative lung complications such as pneumonia. If you smoke, your surgeon will recommend that you stop as soon as you decide to have surgery, so that your lungs will be in the best possible condition. If you suffer from emphysema, chronic bronchitis, asthma, or any other condition for which you are taking medication, be sure to take it in adequate doses, to give yourself your best chance.

Problems related to chemical and fluid composition of your body should be identified and corrected. Dehydration due to lack of fluids can be rapidly corrected with intravenous fluids, but some problems take longer to correct. Malnutrition, so common in chronically ill, hospitalized, elderly, and debilitated persons, is associated with protein deficiency and other chemical imbalances, impaired ability to heal wounds and recover from surgery, and increased susceptibility to infection. A condition of potassium depletion, due most often to diuretic (fluid) pills, chronic diarrhea, or nausea and vomiting, may take days to replace and should be detected as early as possible. If you have diabetes, your blood sugar should be controlled before you enter the hospital. Your physician may start you on multiple doses of short-acting insulin in the so-called perioperative period—that is, before, during, and after surgery.

Significant thyroid dysfunction, acute hepatitis, and liver failure are notorious for causing unacceptably high risk and will require all but the most urgent surgery to be canceled until the condition is improved.

Obesity is often considered a risk factor, and is associated with postoperative blood clots and respiratory and cardiac problems. These risks can be greatly minimized by taking some precautions, so your doctor will probably advise you to abstain from cigarettes for at least four weeks before surgery, and prescribe some form of anticoagulant blood thinner *before* clots develop, monitor your lung and heart function closely, and judiciously use antibiotics to prevent wound infections. If these precautionary measures are followed carefully, the risk of elective surgery in cases of obesity is not much increased. "There is little documented evidence to justify denying surgery to a patient based on body weight alone"(3).

Medication history Your surgeon should be aware of what medications you have been taking. Diuretics may, as we have noted, affect the chemical composition of your body, and may also have effects on your kidney function. If you suddenly stop taking certain blood pressure medications, there may be an abrupt and dangerous rise in blood pressure. If you have recently been treated with cortisone or similar medications, your body's natural ability to cope with the stress of surgery may be seriously impaired.

Classification of risk. Since the 1960s anesthesiologists have regularly used the ASA (American Society of Anesthesiologists) Physical Status Classification to estimate overall surgical risk. This deceptively simple five-level classification is still the best and most widely used predictor of surgical mortality (1).

Class 1 indicates that the patient is in good health but requires surgery for a localized condition not affecting overall health.

Class 2 indicates a patient with some risk factors but no severe health problems. Examples of such risk factors are severe obesity (more than 100 pounds overweight, or more than twice ideal weight), mild emphysema, extreme old age, stable heart disease.

Class 3 patients include those with disease that limits activity but is not incapacitating. Examples are stable angina pectoris, severe diabetes.

Class 4 patients have severe, incapacitating disease. Examples include heart failure, unstable angina, advanced liver or endocrine dysfunction.

Class 5 patients are those who are moribund and have little chance of surviving for twenty-four hours. Surgical risk varies from .01 percent for Class 1, up to 5 percent for Class 3, and greater than 20 percent for class 5. If the surgery is an emergency, the notation E is added to the class designation; this means that the risk is at least twice as great.

Emergency surgery carries a much greater risk than elective, planned surgery. In the case of elective surgery, your physician will have had an opportunity to detect any coexisting conditions or risk factors and correct them or at least be ready to anticipate problems. Your blood pressure will be controlled, your diabetes regulated, and you will be psychologically prepared. Above all, there will be no big surprises during or after the operation.

But in the case of emergency surgery, you and your health may be unknown quantities. You may have alcohol, nicotine, or medication in your body, making your response to anesthesia and surgery unpredictable. You may have food in your stomach that is potentially lethal if you vomit. You may be emotionally traumatized and less than normally able to cope with your illness and medical care. Small wonder, then, that the complication rate of emergency surgery is high.

The best protection, of course, is to prevent the need for emergency surgery. If you have a condition that you know will sooner or later require an operation, get it done sooner, before the condition turns into an emergency. Many injuries which commonly require emergency surgery can be prevented by use of seat belts and other self-protective measures.

Sometimes, of course, the emergency comes out of the blue, and there is no way you can anticipate or prevent it. The danger can nonetheless be minimized. Know your medical history. Know if you have any medical problems. If you haven't had a checkup for years, get one, so that you will know if you have any hidden medical problems. If you have a complicated medical history, have some documentation, especially if you are away from your regular doctor or hospital. The documentation may be in the form of a copy of your medical records, or even an identification bracelet, indicating some particularly important condition, such as diabetes or epilepsy.

If you are taking medication, find out the names and strengths of your medicine. Knowing that you take "a little blue pill" three times a day won't be of much help. A list of medications and dosage could be a lifesaver in some circumstances. If you do have a chronic medical condition, make sure it is well controlled. If, for example, you have high blood pressure controlled by medication, your risk at surgery will be far less than if it is untreated and uncontrolled.

One of the great dangers of emergency surgery is that you might vomit a recently eaten meal, particles of which might obstruct your windpipe. Your doctor can take some preventive steps if you tell him that you have just eaten. Your surgeon may, if possible, delay surgery. If surgery can't be delayed, he or she may try to wash the food out of your stomach, and the anesthesiologist may insert an endotracheal tube into the windpipe so that if you do vomit, food will be kept out.

If you have been drinking, *don't try to hide it*. Alcohol in your blood may impair such all-important reflexes as gagging and coughing and it may change the way you respond to medications. If your surgeon knows, he may try to delay surgery or at least be prepared for the possible complications.

The increased risk of emergency surgery can thus be kept to a minimum.

Provider-related risks.

Once you have selected a surgeon (see Chapter 1), your principal concerns will be the anesthesiologist and the hospital.

Anesthesiologist. The choice of an anesthesiologist will not be yours to make, but it certainly wouldn't hurt to express some interest in the matter. Your surgeon, of course, wants the best possible result, and since he is usually the one who picks the anesthesiologist, he should choose the best possible person. But in some hospitals the anesthesiologist who happens to be on call is the one who will "do" the case, unless your surgeon makes a particular effort to select someone else. If you show great interest in the choice of anesthesiologist, it may heighten your surgeon's interest, too. You might ask who the surgeon favors, what that person's background, training, and experience are. Is it a nurse-anesthetist or a fully trained board certified anesthesiologist? Most importantly, does the surgeon know for sure who the anesthesiologist will be, and has the surgeon worked with that individual before? Is the anesthesia staff at the hospital where you are to have your surgery as good as the staff at other hospitals that your surgeon uses? Your unusual questions may startle or even upset your surgeon a bit, but that is not necessarily bad. You don't want him to think of your case as routine.

Hospital. There are large differences in mortality and complication rates among different hospitals and even among geographic regions. These data are very hard to interpret, however. A higher death rate could mean less skillful care, or it could mean that the patients are sicker to begin with. Or it could mean that the surgeons are willing to take on very serious cases that those with a lower death rate refuse. Some studies indicate that large hospitals do better than small ones, but other studies do not confirm this.

Teaching hospitals closely affiliated with a medical school usually have available the most knowledgeable specialists and most advanced techniques, both especially important in the very complicated and difficult cases. But those hospitals will usually also expose you to inexperienced house staff, the impersonality that goes with large institutions, diffusion of responsibility and limited access to your attending surgeon. The small proprietary, for-profit hospital may be more attentive to your personal needs, and it may be much easier for you to make your wishes known and respected; the customer is always right. Your personal surgeon will probably be intimately involved with the details of your care, and, unlike surgeons in the teaching hospital, he will delegate very little. But in case of a crisis, such a hospital may not be able to muster all the needed resources. The nonprofit community hospital often has features that are intermediate between these extremes. These comments are generalizations, to which of course, there are many exceptions.

Choice of hospital then depends on personal preference, the kind of services you anticipate the need for, and, above all, perhaps, the recommendation of your surgeon, whose direct experience with the hospital should make his choice an informed one.

It is clear, though, that for certain operations that require skillful teamwork, hospitals with a high volume have better results. Open-heart surgery—as for replacement of a defective valve—is such a procedure. It looks so simple, the way the surgeon cuts away the diseased valve and sews in the mechanical prosthesis. It takes no remarkable dexterity or artistry. What it takes is remarkable, quiet, effortless teamwork. For while the surgeon is sewing in the valve, the anesthesiologist is monitoring every vital life function and carefully controlling the patient's body temperature, which has been brought very low to minimize the brain's need for oxygen. The patient's heart has been stopped, and its function taken over by an elaborate heart-lung device, which is run by the pump team. The pump team must do exactly the right things at the right time. The patient will die on the table or later on of complications if there is a mechanical problem or human error. When the new valve is in place, the anesthesia is lightened, the body temperature is slowly raised, the heart restarted, the heart-lung machine disconnected, the necessary blood transfused, the appropriate medications injected. This must be done with no hesitation; just a word here and a grunt there. That is the kind of teamwork that can be developed and maintained only by a group that perform 100 to 200 such operations a year.

Complications

So far we have been considering the risk of dying. Complications are another, albeit lesser risk. One cause of complications is, of course, faulty surgical technique: the wrong tube tied off; the bowel accidentally punctured; the knot that comes loose; the break in sterile technique. All these can lead to postoperative complications.

Some complications are caused by circumstances beyond the surgeon's control: the appendix already burst before surgery; emphysema; the compromised circulation of the diabetic; the weakened resistance of the malnourished. These too can lead to postoperative complications.

Each operation has its unique complications, but there are some that may occur after almost any major surgery; I will discuss some of the more common ones.

Contaminations. Surgical cases are often divided into two categories: "clean" and "contaminated" (often called "dirty"). Which of these categories your case falls into usually depends on the nature of your illness or the

Surgery

circumstances of your injury, factors beyond the control of you and your surgeon. In a clean case the surgery does not involve infected material or tissue. Replacement of a hip joint destroyed by arthritis, for example, is a clean case. Except for the skin, which is disinfected, the surgery will not contact tissue that is expected to harbor any infection. A wound infection in a clean case occurs only 2 to 4 percent of the time. Such a complication in a normally clean case causes much concern. It implies a break in sterile technique, which the infection-control nurse or hospital epidemiologist will try to pinpoint and correct.

A contaminated case is one involving already infected tissue, such as drainage of an abscess, exploratory surgery in a case of peritonitis, or treatment of a contaminated wound such as a compound leg fracture. In cases of emergency surgery on the intestine, the wound infection rate may be as high as 60 percent (4). In clean cases wound infections are avoided by meticulous sterile technique. In contaminated cases wound infection is avoided or controlled by use of antibiotics, drainage of abscesses, and removal of dead tissue.

Pneumonia is another common and feared complication of surgery. Part of the body's natural resistance to pneumonia is the ability to cough foreign matter out of the bronchial tubes and windpipe. After surgery, expecially surgery of the chest or abdomen, it is difficult to take a deep breath, and it hurts to cough. If, on top of that, you have emphysema, bronchitis, a cigarette habit, or severe obesity, the risk of penumonia is much greater. To make matters worse, pneumonia acquired in the hospital is sometimes caused by the particularly tough microbes that have learned how to survive in that antibiotic-laden atmosphere. To prevent postoperative pneumonia, ask your doctor about breathing exercises to perform before the surgery, avoid cigarettes for two months (4a) and, before you enter the hospital, if you have asthma or bronchitis, take adequate medication.

Blood clots in the leg veins (deep vein thrombosis—DVT) occur commonly after surgery. In response to injury—and surgery is an injury—the blood's natural tendency to clot increases. Furthermore, you are immobilized first by anesthesia and later by bedrest, so that the circulation in your legs is slowed. These two factors account, in part, for the frequent occurrence of DVT. Deep vein thrombosis can cause pain and swelling of the legs, but it can also occur without any symptoms. But whether it causes symptoms or not, a piece of the clot can break off and float through the bloodstream to the lungs. Such clots in the lungs can be fatal and are, in fact, one of the major causes of postoperative deaths. If you are very obese, have heart failure, are taking contraceptive pills, have cancer or a leg injury, the risk of DVT is high.

Experts agree that deep-vein thrombosis can often be prevented by wearing pressurized stockings (like a spacesuit) or by taking anticoagulant blood thinners. These measures are not universally used, however, because of habit, expense, inconvenience, and the fear of postoperative bleeding. In the high risk situations noted above, however, some sort of preventive measures should be undertaken.

Shock. A serious postoperative complication is shock, which is manifested by a blood pressure so low that there is insufficient blood flow to the brain, kidneys, heart muscle, and other vital organs. This complication can be fatal if not promptly diagnosed and treated. Postoperative shock may be due to prolonged effects of anesthesia or oversedation. In such cases the surgeon need only tide the patient over with appropriate medications and intravenous fluids until the effect wears off. But other causes of shock may require more aggressive treatment. If there has been more bleeding during surgery than was realized, or if there is hidden bleeding in the postoperative period, blood transfusion may be lifesaving. If the shock is due to a heart attack precipitated by the stress of surgery, appropriate medical care and monitoring in an intensive care unit are critical. Another common cause of shock is infection, especially if bacteria have entered into the bloodstream. It is vital that this complication be quickly recognized, because it is commonly fatal if antibiotics are not promptly administered.

Postoperative kidney failure has several possible causes, all of which require different treatment, so a correct diagnosis is essential. If the blood pressure has fallen below a critical level for a critical period of time, either before or during surgery, the kidneys may shut down and cease to function. This shutdown may be partial, in which case there is a temporary decrease in the amount of urine produced, or may be prolonged and severe, in which case the patient may need an artificial kidney until recovery occurs (which it almost always does). Treatment of this kind of kidney failure is like a difficult balancing act. If not enough fluids are administered, the kidney shutdown will be intensified. If too much fluid is administered, the kidneys may become overwhelmed and allow fluid to accumulate in excess. This excess may overtax the heart and cause heart failure. An internist or nephrologist (kidney specialist) will often be summoned to assist in the treatment of these cases.

Some medications can cause kidney failure. These include some antibiotics (especially those known as aminoglycosides) that are especially useful in the treatment of infections of the gallbladder, intestines, and pelvic organs. Trouble can usually, but not always, be avoided by monitoring kidney function and measuring the concentration of the antibiotic in the blood.

Another class of drugs that may cause kidney failure is the nonsteroidal anti-inflammatory class, which includes such common and otherwise excellent medications as ibuprofen (Motrin, Advil, Medipren, and others), indomethacin (Indocin) and many others. These medications should be

Surgery 123

avoided in case of preexisting kidney impairment, heart failure, or dehydration.

If kidney failure occurs in the postoperative period, the patient's medication record must be immediately and critically reviewed, for if the offending medication is continued, irreversible destruction of the kidneys may occur.

Catheter problems. If a patient has a catheter tube in the bladder and this gets blocked by blood clots or a mechanical problem, urine output will cease and kidney failure may be wrongly diagnosed. Such a blockage can be detected by flushing the catheter with an irrigating fluid. If the fluid flows freely, there is no blockage; if there is a blockage, the catheter must be replaced. A blockage must be recognized promptly, because if it is allowed to persist, true kidney failure will ensue.

Perhaps the most common urinary tract complication is bladder or kidney infection caused by the catheters so often needed during or after surgery. If the catheter is still in place, fever is the most common symptom. If the infection shows up after the catheter has been removed, the usual symptoms include frequent, burning urination, fever, and back pain. The diagnosis is usually made by examining the urine. Cure requires the use of antibiotics, lots of fluids, and removal of the catheter, if it is still present, as soon as possible.

Gastrointestinal problems. One of the most miserable complications of surgery is distension or blockage of part of the gastrointestinal tract. When this complication occurs, it is usually after abdominal surgery. Diabetes and chemical imbalances such as a lack of potassium predispose to this complication. After surgery the bowel frequently becomes paralyzed for a period of time. As a result, swallowed air, gases produced by the bacteria normally in the intestines, and the fluid produced by the stomach and intestines, are not expelled or absorbed. This causes distension, sometimes massive, of the stomach or parts of the intestine. The patient experiences severe pain, vomiting, and even shock. The treatment consists of passing a tube through the nose, or mouth, and down into the stomach and beyond, to reach the area that is distended. Gentle suction can decompress the bowel. After a few days, the intestines recover, and the tube can be removed. Rarely, though, a mechanical blockage may occur; in that case another operation may be required to relieve the obstruction. If you have intestinal surgery, don't be surprised or distressed if you wake up with a gastric tube already in place; your surgeon may be preventing trouble.

Neuro/psychiatric and emotional disorders sometimes occur in the postoperative period. The symptoms vary in intensity, from an exaggeration of the normal anxiety and concern about body image to a life-threatening, frankly psychotic loss of touch with reality. Sometimes, inexplicably, the symptoms begin after two or three days of what seems to be a perfectly smooth postoperative period. Feelings of depression, concern about bodily appearance and function, sleeplessness and mild confusion are common. Severe cases, in which the patient becomes delirious and out of touch with reality, occur in less than 0.5 percent of cases of ordinary operations such as abdominal surgery, but are much more common after other kinds, especially open-heart surgery. Emotional and physical factors, usually inextricably intertwined, contribute. Physical and chemical factors must be important because the most severe of these problems occur in the elderly, and those with pre-existing memory loss, serious illness of any kind or a history of chemical substance dependency. Depending on the severity of the symptoms, simple reassurance, the use of psychoactive medications, or the assistance of a psychiatrist may be needed.

Psychological factors may be just as important, and this is an area where you can take steps to protect yourself, if you are to have surgery. Don't put your head in the sand. Denial as a psychologic defense mechanism has its place, but it doesn't work well as a preparation for surgery. Postoperative reality will come barging through, and you will find yourself unprepared.

If you can't tolerate pain and are afraid of it, tell your surgeon. Postoperative pain can be controlled. To avoid drug toxicity and dependency, however, surgeons tend to use the smallest amount of pain reliever and so sometimes err on the side of too little. Tell your surgeon not to do that—he or she will probably take heed.

If the surgery involves your sexual organs, find out *ahead of time* what the effects on your sex life may be. Talk to your doctor, talk to your sex partner. If your surgery is expected to be disfiguring, plan for plastic surgery, so that when you first face your scar, you will already know what steps will be taken to restore your appearance.

Find out how long you will be out of work, and prepare your boss, coworkers, or clients for your absence. Make arrangements for child care, payment of bills, and other household responsibilities. Check the details of your health insurance coverage so that you will get the maximum allowance and will know what part of the bill you will have to pay out of pocket.

Above all, don't be alone. Don't be a martyr. Organize your troops, mobilize your support system. Have the people with you that you can count on, to hold your hand, to love you even if you look and feel a mess. And it doesn't hurt to have an advocate on hand. Nurses and the myriad of other health-care workers devote themselves to the care of patients, but sometimes they are overworked and understaffed and so may not know of some unmet needs you have. A tactful, confident significant-other can rectify this and make sure that the staff knows that there is someone who cares, and is keeping an eye on things. If all goes well, as it usually does, in no time you will be able to fend quite well for yourself.

Blood transfusion may be another source of trouble. You may need a blood transfusion before surgery if you have been bleeding or are severely anemic; you may need it during or after surgery to replace blood loss. Blood as such, known as whole blood, is rarely used in transfusion nowadays. Blood is usually separated into several components: red blood cells, which are the oxygen-carrying component; plasma, the fluid and "volume" component, which can be frozen and stored for a long time; platelets, which are necessary for normal clotting; numerous other less often used components including white blood cells, and subdivisions of the plasma that contain various clot-promoting factors and antibodies.

Ordinarily "blood" transfused in connection with surgery is the red blood cell component, called packed red blood cells (PRBC). The red blood cells are much more concentrated than in normal blood—hence, "packed." If in addition to a need for oxygen-carrying red cells, there is insufficient volume of blood, it is customary to give a salt solution, or, if the situation is acute or critical, plasma, along with the packed red cells.

As we have previously noted, in the early days of transfusion therapy, a transfusion reaction, due to incompatibility of the blood, was the great fear. Modern methods of blood typing make such reactions almost unheard of. When they do occur, it is almost always because there has been a mixup: The patient was given the wrong person's blood. Few things in clinical medicine are as hazardous as giving one person's blood to someone else. Because of this, hospitals have a ritual for double and triple checking the label on the blood against the patient's identification bracelet, thus minimizing the possibility of an error. There are some diseases and medications that make blood typing difficult, and in those cases minor reactions may occur in spite of all best efforts.

The hazard of blood transfusion that has had the most attention recently is, of course, the transmission of AIDS. There have been many cases. Among patients who have hemophilia, the bleeding tendency that requires the administration of a blood product that is derived from combining the clotting factors of multiple donors, over 70 percent have been infected with the AIDS virus. This complication is one of the great tragedies in the history of medical treatment. However, since the advent, in 1983, of tests for the AIDS virus antibody, the risk of getting infected by blood transfusion has been essentially eliminated. The risk is at most 1 in 100,000 units transfused, and more likely 1 in 1 million.

Much more frequent, unfortunately, is the transmission of a kind of hepatitis known as non-A, non-B hepatitis. Hepatitis A and B are the well known, common forms of hepatitis. There are tests that can detect the presence of the viruses that cause them; if it is present, the blood is not accepted. There is another form of hepatitis, however, which is neither A nor

B. The cause of this hepatitis is not known, and there is no test for it, so it cannot be kept out of the blood supply. The risk is minimized if the blood is from volunteer rather than paid donors, and if the blood is screened carefully for the presence of any trace of liver disease. This is done by testing for an abnormal increase of liver enzymes in the blood. But even so, a 1987 report (5) showed that for each single unit of blood transfused, the recipient had a 2 percent chance of getting hepatitis. Since most transfusions are for two to six units, the usual risk varies between 4 percent and 12 percent. Although three fourths of the time there are no symptoms at first, over half of the patients who get hepatitis go on to develop chronic liver disease. Such liver disease can be serious and even fatal.

The best way to avoid the risk is to avoid having a transfusion. You should let your surgeon know that you are concerned about this issue. He may be surprised, or even uncomfortable, but it may stay his hand if, later on, the need for a transfusion is marginal. It would also be helpful to know that the blood bank from which the blood will be drawn uses only volunteer donors and checks the blood for abnormal levels of liver enzymes.

Autologous transfusion—using the patient's own blood—is another way to avoid transfusion hepatitis without giving up any of the benefits of a transfusion. This should definitely be discussed with your doctor. In the case of autologous transfusion, you go to the blood bank as much as three weeks before surgery and "donate" one or more pints of blood. This blood is stored, and, if you need a transfusion at the time of the surgery, you are given your own blood back. Assuming that there is no mix-up with the labeling and administering of the blood, this will avoid completely the risk of transfusion hepatitis.

Unnecessary Surgery

Unnecessary surgery is a difficult topic, because, although there is no good or widely accepted definition of unnecessary surgery (6), the term carries implications of poor care, dangerous practices, greed, and exploitation.

A number of observations support the idea that surgery is sometimes performed when it need not be or, indeed, ought not be. Review of surgical specimens show that sometimes perfectly healthy organs are surgically removed. The number of operations varies from region to region within the country. The number of operations in Britain is much smaller than for a comparable population in the United States. Patients who get care from an HMO have less surgery than their counterparts with conventional health insurance. When patients are required to have a second opinion before surgery, 7 to 25 percent of the time the second surgeon does not recommend surgery. Operations most frequently cited in studies of unnecessary surgery include hysterectomy, gallbladder surgery, coronary artery bypass, and carotid endarterectomy (for relieving blockage of the carotid arteries in the neck).

Let us consider some practices that might be considered unnecessary surgery. The surgeon may deliberately and knowingly perform operations for which there is no medical need. This may be for financial gain or perverse personal motives. I don't think anyone knows how often this happens. My personal experience suggests that it is rare. But it does occur. Your defense against this risk is, of course, in your choice of surgeon. How to choose a good surgeon has been discussed elsewhere in this book. A surgeon respected by his peers, recommended by another physician you trust, who operates in a good hospital, is unlikely to be the sort who does this kind of unnecessary surgery.

Sometimes there is no objective measure of the need for, or appropriateness of, surgery. Consider again the painful hip joint, destroyed by arthritis. If it hurts too much, or is too disabling, surgery is called for. But how to measure too much pain, and how much disability is too much? Predictably, honest opinions will differ. The surgeon who recommends surgery will be influenced by his values and his perception of the patient's discomfort. Is he recommending unnecessary surgery? Another surgeon will perceive things differently and so, perhaps, make a different recommendation.

In a 1987 study (7) it was found that a second opinion before coronary artery bypass resulted in a 50 percent reduction in surgery. What is one to make of this? There is a suggestion that the patients who sought a second opinion had doubtful cases to begin with or were individuals who had a bias against surgical treatment. But that, certainly, is not a complete explanation. As we noted earlier, the risk/benefit ratio for CABG is, in many cases, largely unknown. In such circumstances the physician recommending for or against surgery will be influenced by his personal experience, the availability of consultants, the availability of a hospital and cardiac surgery program, and the standards of his particular medical community. Similar considerations may help explain the variance in surgery rates in different localities and communities.

If you want to avoid "unnecessary" surgery, understand what nonsurgical treatments are available, and try those first. So-called conservative measures might include medications, splints or other devices, injections, physical therapy, diet, or life-style changes. If conservative treatment fails but you are still unsure about surgery, consider a second opinion. If you trust your surgeon but want reassurance about the recommendation for surgery, ask him to refer you, preferably to someone with whom he is not directly associated. Or you can ask your primary-care physician for a referral. Or you can start from scratch and get a completely independent opinion.

Getting a second opinion is not, however, without hazards. If the second opinion is the same as the first, this will be very reassuring—if both opinions agree with your own. But if you didn't accept the first recommendation for surgery, and the second one fails to convince you, too, your anxiety about the matter will simply escalate. If you have made up your mind not to have surgery, then have the courage of that conviction. It is probably better than shopping around until you find a doctor who agrees with you.

If the first and second opinions are different, you will, of course, be in a difficult situation. How can you know that the second opinion is better than the first? If the second opinion confirms your desire to refuse surgery, you may accept it. But if you were seeking confirmation of the first opinion, your uncertainty will only increase, and you will, in the end, have to make up your own mind. So, while second opinions, popular with some insurance companies and government agencies, may decrease the surgery rate and decrease "unnecessary" surgery and decrease costs, they are not always helpful to the individual when decision time comes around.

BENEFITS

After considering this great catalog of surgical risks, why would anyone willingly "go under the knife?" What benefits could outweigh such risks?

The first, of course, is the immediate saving of life: if you have suffered grievous injury; if your broken bone end is protruding through the skin; if you are bleeding internally; if your shattered rib has punctured and collapsed your lung; if a bullet has perforated your colon; if the aneurism in your aorta has started to bleed into your flank. In such emergency situations, pray that a surgeon and a surgical nurse and a lab technician are on hand. Never mind now the consent form or the risk of blood transfusion; it is time to go to the OR. Saving a life is the great benefit for you, and the great reward to the hardy physicians willing to take the challenge.

The next great benefit is, of course, cure. So many of life's ills are incurable. They may be controllable, they may be endurable, but they are not curable. But surgeons often cure. Are your gallstones making you sweat with pain? Is your slipped disk paralyzing your leg? Are you suffering the relentless cramps of intestinal obstruction? Is the shadow of a cataract darkening your world? Is the cancer on your skin slowly growing? Has your prostate gland made the passage of urine, so long taken for granted, a difficult and humiliating effort? Your surgeon can cure you.

Sometimes cure is not possible but relief is. CABG surgery and bypass surgery for blocked arteries in the legs may at times eliminate the pain even though there is persisting and severe blockage of the remaining blood vessels.

Surgery

A joint deformed by rheumatoid arthritis can be straightened even though, overall, the arthritis is unaffected. Laser surgery of the retina injured by diabetes may temporarily restore sight or halt worsening. If the relief provided by surgery is expected to be only a brief respite from a disease such as incurable cancer, this kind of surgery is sometimes called palliative. Cutting a nerve to kill the pain, performing a colostomy to bypass the rectal obstruction, pinning a hip fractured by a bone tumor are examples of this kind of surgery: relief without cure.

Surgery may be performed to prevent illness. This is sometimes called prophylactic surgery. It protects you from future harm. You may have gallstones quietly floating around in your gallbladder, not bothering you. Better have them out, you may be advised, to avoid another gallbladder attack, or even worse, an infection in the gallbladder and liver. Better fix the hernia before it strangulates. Remove the colon polyp before it turns malignant. Repair the aneurism before it bursts.

Surgery may be reconstructive and restorative. Surgeons can remove disfiguring scars, straighten a congenitally twisted foot, restore the pleasing contour marred by a mastectomy.

It takes few words to describe the benefits: Surgery can save you, cure you, relieve you, protect you, and restore you.

SURGICAL TECHNIQUES

Conventional surgical techniques are a commonplace of our culture. Sterile gowns and gloves, aseptic technique, the scalpel, the suture, the hemostat, and the sponge count, are known to every schoolchild. This is still the surgeon's craft and skill: to control the bleeding; to tie the perfect knot; to join perfectly the cut ends of an artery; to know how much to cut away and how much to leave; to decide, on the spot, without consultation or discussion, what must be done and have the ability to do it.

Endoscopic surgery. Conventional surgery is nowadays often complemented or even replaced by endoscopic surgery. An endoscope is a fiberoptic tube that transmits a brilliant and sharp image no matter how many twists and turns it has to traverse. It gives the user an endoscopic, or inside view, of breathtaking clarity. There are endoscopes for looking into the colon or stomach, the joints, abdominal cavity, the urinary bladder, the inside of arteries and veins, other cavities and orifices. It is possible to snare, cut, burn, or freeze tissue through the endoscope. Polyps can be removed, veins injected, blood vessels burned, ulcers frozen, joint cartilage removed or repaired, Fallopian tubes tied.

Balloon angioplasty. Surgery on blood vessels has been greatly aided by the recent advent of "balloon surgery," which opens up blocked arteries. This procedure is most commonly applied to the coronary arteries and is known as percutaneous transluminal coronary angioplasty (PTCA). A deflated balloon, attached to a hollow tube, is passed through a small incision in the skin (percutaneous), then into the main artery of the leg, then passed through (trans) the channel (lumin) to the blocked coronary artery. When the balloon is at the narrow place of the artery (angio), it is inflated and so stretches open (plasty) the narrow or blocked segment. Arteries to the kidney and some other blood vessels can be similarly opened up. PTCA can sometimes take the place of open heart or other major surgery.

Lasers. An even more dramatic new technique is the use of Light Amplification by Stimulated Emission of Radiation: the laser. When certain substances are "stimulated" by, for example, high voltage electric current, the atoms of that substance become energized and begin to radiate photons. They glow. Amplification of such stimulated radiation emissions produces the laser beam. Laser beams can cut through three-inch thick steel; they can reach the moon. They can be controlled precisely enough to remove a tumor wrapped around an artery.

The light of a laser differs from ordinary light in three important ways. Ordinary light is composed of light of many wavelengths (colors); it radiates in all directions and so disperses; the light waves are noncoherent—the individual waves are out of phase with each other. Light from a laser is monochromatic—it is composed entirely of one wavelength or color; all the rays are parallel, so the laser light does not disperse; the light waves are coherent—they are all in phase.

As a surgical instrument, the laser has remarkable properties. Unlike a scalpel which can spread infection, the laser, being just a beam of light, is always sterile. Furthermore the heat of the laser sterilizes already infected tissues. A contaminated wound can be converted into a clean wound. When a scalpel cuts across capillaries and small arteries, bleeding ensues. When the laser cuts, it simultaneously cauterizes and seals the blood vessels. The laser beam can be directed into spaces ordinarily difficult to reach—deep into the ear, for example, or the channel in an artery. And of course the laser, unlike any mechanical instrument, can go through the transparent part of the eye to reach the retina. The laser can be used to cut, to cauterize, and to "weld" tissue together. That is how a detached retina is reattached to the back of the eye.

Microscope surgery. Surgeons sometimes use an operating microscope to dissect or repair nerves and blood vessels too small to be seen adequately with the unaided eye. The sutures are finer than a hair, and sometimes mechanical devices are used because the necessary manipulations are too subtle to be accomplished freehand. The microscope is sometimes used for surgery on the eye, brain, spinal cord, hand, Fallopian tubes, testicle, and other organs.

Ultrasound. Ultrasound energy can be used to break up stones. Before the advent of ultrasound surgery, if you had a large kidney stone that was causing trouble, a major operation was in store for you. A large incision in your flank was required to expose the kidney, which itself had to be widely opened to allow removal of the stone. A long hospital stay was required even if you were lucky enough to escape any complications. Now your urologist can pass an ultrasound probe through an incision less than an inch long, right into your kidney and painlessly destroy the stone totally or suction out a few remaining fragments. This is commonly done as an outpatient procedure.

Shock waves. Extracorporeal lithotripsy is the name for the new shock wave treatment for kidney stones. This method requires no incision at all. Instead of an operating room table, there is a tub in which you are immersed and put to sleep. Electric sparks generate powerful shock waves in the water, which are focused on your kidney stones. The soft tissues of your body just vibrate but the brittle stone bursts into tiny pieces, which can later pass out through the urine. No incision, no sutures or staples, no wound infections.

KINDS OF SURGERY

In this final section I will mention some of the newer developments in surgery. Since this subject is too large to cover systematically, I have chosen a few topics of particular interest or timeliness.

General surgery. General surgery deals with most surgical problems that do not require a surgical subspecialist. These problems include most injuries, hernia repairs, gastrointestinal operations, and many cancer operations. More and more procedures, including many hernia repairs, are being done outpatient. Newer developments include the use of sophisticated stapling devices for joining the cut ends of bowel, more accurate diagnostic tests, including CAT scan and ultrasound, use of lasers and use of autologous transfusions.

Recent developments have caused much discussion about one of the oldest and most common operations: removal of the diseased gallbladder and the stones it contains. For years it was taught that symptomless gallstones, especially in a diabetic person, should be removed a soon as possible to prevent future complications. Recent careful studies have shown that such prophylactic surgery is not necessary. Many patients will never require surgery and those that do later on are not harmed by the delay.

Researchers have discovered that certain medications can dissolve stones and that shock wave therapy can break them up. The problem with these treatments is that in the process of dissolving or breaking up the stones, they get smaller. Smaller stones can sometimes cause more trouble than large ones, because they are more likely to move around. And in any case, gallbladder stones tend to recur so that the medication has to be taken indefinitely or the shock wave therapy done repeatedly. So conventional surgery is still the best treatment except for exceptional circumstances when surgery is impossible or extremely risky.

Cardiovascular surgery. Surgery of the heart and blood vessels continues to advance rapidly. We have already discussed the most common heart surgery, CABG or coronary artery bypass graft. The mortality rate at many institutions is now less than 1 percent. Even complicated and previously lethal congenital heart lesions can often be repaired, and replacement of defective heart valves is almost routine. Mechanical heart valves all have the major drawback of tending to form clots, however, so valves removed from the hearts of pigs continue to be used. Their major disadvantage is that they wear out after a few years. Because of these problems, surgeons are trying harder to repair rather than replace damaged valves.

A common affliction of elderly cigarette smokers is blockage of the arteries to the legs. If the blockage cannot be removed by balloon angioplasty or laser surgery, veins from the leg or arm, or synthetic tubes are often used to bypass the blockage and so save limbs. The dangerous ballooning of a weakened segment of artery, known as an aneurism, can often be repaired by replacing the aneurism with a synthetic artery.

Neurosurgery. Neurosurgery is one of the super high-tech surgical areas. Lasers, stereotactic probes, and operating microscopes are now commonly used. The cure of malignant brain tumors usually remains beyond the reach of even these sophisticated techniques, but significant palliation is often possible. Head-injury patients have a much better chance of recovery thanks to some new treatments, but removal of blood clots from the surface of the brain and control of bleeding remain key tasks for neurosurgeons. The repair of aneurisms of the brain, drainage of abscesses, and relief of pressure due to fluid buildup are areas of considerable success. Surgery on the spine has made great progress, too, thanks to the microscope and laser. Surgery for slipped disk has been greatly aided by CAT scans. At times surgery can be avoided by injecting the disk with enzymes that dissolve the tissue that is pressing on the nerve.

Orthopedic surgery. Orthopedists routinely replace worn out hip joints and have the patients walking around the wards within forty-eight hours. Even knees and some smaller joints can now be replaced with a high success rate. The use of high-tech glues to keep the artificial joints in place have solved some old problems. Infection remains a great fear and still occurs in spite of meticulous technique, operating rooms with "laminar airflow," and new antibiotics. Arthroscopic surgery allows outpatient procedures and rapid recovery of function even for badly deranged knee and shoulder joints.

Cancer surgery. The kinds of operations surgeons perform for the treatment of the patient with cancer are determined by the surgeon's ideas about the nature of the disease, and his technical ability to perform the surgery. Both these factors continue to undergo rapid change. When cancer is considered a disease that begins in one discrete place and gradually grows and extends its margins, the logical surgical procedure is to remove the cancer and the surrounding tissue. If the operation fails to cure, the temptation is to remove ever larger amounts of tissue. Breast cancer surgery is an example of this approach. In the nineteenth and even eighteenth century, breast cancer patients underwent mastectomy. The high rate of failure, even when the tumor was small, encouraged surgeons to do ever more extensive operations. This led to the radical mastectomy developed by Halsted at the turn of the century, and it is still with us. With the advent of technological progress that made it possible for patients to survive ultraradical surgery, mastectomy was further extended. The 1950s and 1960s saw the so-called extended radical mastectomy in which the surgeon removes the entire breast, skin and all, the pectoral muscles underneath the breast, half of the breastbone, the lymph glands adjacent to and behind the breast bone, parts of four ribs, part of the covering of the lung, and all the tissue and lymph glands in the armpit. A skin graft larger than a dinner plate is laid upon the exposed ribs to replace the missing skin. The patient is left with a chest like a washboard, a weak and swollen arm, and a long and difficult recovery. That was also the era of the ultraradical surgery: removal of half or even more of the face; removal of all the pelvic organs including the sexual organs, the bladder, and the rectum with drainage of feces and urine through openings in the abdominal wall; removal of an entire leg, hip, and half of the pelvis. Modern techniques allowed the patients to survive the surgery but only infrequently did they survive the disease, which was not eradicated by even these drastic methods.

For decades the radical mastectomy (with some variations) continued to be the only "curative" operation performed for breast cancer, even though breast cancer mortality did not decrease, and even though it had been noted since ancient times (Celsus, 1st century A.D.) that sometimes surgery only seemed to make the cancer spread. Such observations were ignored or scorned. But in recent years, thanks in part to the courage of surgeon George Crile and others, an objective examination of the failure of radical operations has led to great changes in the surgical approach.

The cancer illness is now viewed as a dynamic interaction between the patient's resistance and the tumor's ability to overcome or circumvent that resistance. When resistance is high, new cancer cells are killed off as quickly as they appear. When resistance is somewhat impaired, a cancer may develop, but it may be held at bay for a long period. When resistance is low, the cancer cells rapidly spread throughout the body, even before the "primary" lump is detected. That concept tends to negate the rationale for ultraradical surgery.

Another factor influencing the surgical approach is availability of more and better data showing that the cure rate does not necessarily rise as the surgery becomes more radical. The third element is the rising influence of the consumer and feminist movements, which see traditional surgical practice as insensitive, sexist, authoritarian, and self-serving.

As a result of these forces, cancer surgery is now likely to be tailored to individual needs and wishes, to be more conservative, and to be combined with other treatment methods including low-dose chemotherapy and safe levels of radiation therapy. If you are advised to have surgery for breast cancer, or indeed any cancer, you have the right to ask your surgeon to sit down and discuss your options with regard to the type and extent of surgery and compare all forms of surgery to all forms of nonsurgical treatment.

In the case of breast cancer, the greatest recent advance has been to separate the diagnostic biopsy from the treatment decision. Previously, if cancer was suspected, you were taken to the operating room, and a biopsy was done. The pathologist would freeze the biopsy tissues and quickly examine it under the microscope while you were still under anesthesia. If cancer was found, your surgeon would do a mastectomy. You wouldn't know ahead of time if you were going to have a simple biopsy or a radical mastectomy.

It is now widely accepted that in the case of a suspicious lump in the breast, or a suspicious image on the mammogram X ray, the first step is to do a biopsy (which may remove the tumor entirely if it is small) to see if the suspicious area is a cancer or benign. The pathologist can carefully study and test the preserved biopsy tissue and, if necessary, obtain consultation and another opinion, to make the most accurate possible diagnosis. You can then discuss the results of the biopsy with your surgeon and decide what further treatment to have. If the biopsy showed cancer, you will probably be advised to choose between removal of the whole breast and removal of the tumor only with subsequent X-ray treatment of the remaining breast tissue. Although there is still uncertainty and some controversy, it appears that both methods may be equally effective in preventing a recurrence.

Another important consideration is the spread of cancer to the lymph glands in the armpit. This can only be determined by a second, minor operation, in which some of the lymph glands are removed and examined by a pathologist. If the nodes show cancer, chemotherapy will usually be advised in addition to the mastectomy or radiation treatment. If, after due consideration of the pros and cons, you choose mastectomy, the discussion should include the issue of breast reconstruction, which can be started immediately or after some delay.

Eye surgery. I have already made reference to some of the modern surgical methods of dealing with derangements of that incredible round marvel, the eye. The cornea, like a watch crystal but alive and literally breathing, is the first layer through which light must traverse if the eye is to "see." If the cornea is badly out of shape, eyeglasses, or contact lenses can often help; if not, "radial keratotomy" can be performed. The cornea is carved up like a pie, the pieces realigned and a new, better shaped cornea results. Beyond the cornea is the lens, also a living marvel that changes shape to keep vision sharply focused. If it becomes clouded by age or diabetes, it can be extracted, and a plastic lens implanted in its place. Sometimes the lens capsule, necessarily left behind, becomes clouded. A zap of the laser will remove the veil. If pressure within the eye builds up because of glaucoma, the laser can be used to drill a tiny hole to let the fluid drain out. Behind the lens is the clear jelly of the interior of the eyeball, and against the far wall is the retina. These structures, too, can often be repaired or protected thanks to the meticulous work of these most particular specialists.

Urologic surgery. We have already considered some aspects of surgery for kidney stones. Surgery for the obstructing enlargement of the prostate gland, so common in late middle life, can be treated with a high degree of success and a very low complication rate thanks to the refinement of transurethral surgery—surgery performed through the penis. Cancer of the urinary tract is a much more difficult problem. Surgical cure of cancer of the prostate, bladder, or kidneys is often not possible because the disease tends to spread early and be detected late. Use of an ultrasound rectal probe to "see" the prostate may allow earlier detection of cancer and perhaps more frequent cure. Male impotence is now being treated with some ingenious implanted devices that the owner can inflate or collapse at will. The medical literature is full of intriguing reports of marvelous accomplishments in this area, at least from the technical standpoint. But I suspect that the long-term benefits for love and happiness have yet to be adequately assessed.

Transplantation. Transplantation surgery is the new frontier, it is the space travel of surgery, and it has been fascinating humankind for centuries. The most famous account of antiquity is the miracle of Cosmas and Damian in the third or fourth century A.D. As the story goes, Cosmas was a physician and Damian a surgeon; together they attended an elderly parishioner with a gangrenous, cancerous leg. They sawed off the diseased member and replaced it with a fresh black leg of a Moor, who had died and been buried that same day in the cemetery of St. Peter's. This tale foretells not only the success of transplantation, but also the necessary joining of medical and surgical science.

The first requisite for successful transplantation is, of course, the matter of surgical technique. We have already noted how anesthesia, antisepsis, and blood transfusion ushered in the era of modern surgery. Transplantation surgery had to await the additional technical advance of vascular anastomosis—i.e., the successful joining together of severed blood vessels. With this development, transplantation of major organs, and reattachment of severed limbs, became a technical reality. But survival of the transplanted organ was most often not possible because of the rejection phenomenon. The recipient's body mounts a fierce attack against the foreign tissue and regularly destroys the graft except in special circumstances—like a graft from an identical twin. Truly successful transplantation had to await the development of methods to suppress the rejection. An array of techniques including the use of hormones, radiation, and immunosuppressive drugs have had a large measure of success but at the price of considerable toxicity. Better methods will surely be developed.

Kidney transplantation is no longer exotic; certainly it doesn't make the front pages. It works; it restores normal life to those who less than two decades ago would have died. Thousands of renal transplant patients make their normal daily rounds through life.

Heart transplantation has not reached such a pinnacle but it, too, has a high immediate success rate, and five years of life of reasonable quality is no rarity. Finding donor hearts is, obviously, much more of a problem than finding donor kidneys. Indeed, the donor problem may turn out to be the limiting factor in heart transplantation. It is possible that a truly successfully mechanical heart may yet replace transplantation. The issue is, I believe, still in doubt.

Still in the realm of the experimental is transplantation of lungs, liver, and pancreas.

And in the realm of fantasy is transplantation of the brain: Who would be the donor and who the recipient in that case? These are not questions you are likely to face anytime soon.

6

SUBSTANCE ABUSE
Marigail Wynne, M.D.

You Have Asked Me About Whiskey. Alright. This is Just How I Stand on the Question. . . . If when you say whiskey, you mean the devils' brew, the poison scourge, the bloody monster that defiles innocents, yeah, literally takes the bread from the mouths of little children; if you mean the evil drink that topples the Christian man and woman from pinnacles of righteous, gracious living into the bottomless pit of degradation and despair, shame and helplessness and hopelessness, then certainly I am against it with all my power.

But, if when you say whiskey, you mean the oil of conversation, the philosophic wine, the stuff that is consumed when good fellows get together, that puts a song in their hearts and laughter on their lips and the warm glow of contentment in their eyes; if you mean the drink that enables a man to magnify his joy, and his happiness, and to forget, if only for a little while, life's great tragedies, heartbreak and sorrows, if you mean the drink, the sale of which pours into our treasuries untold billions of dollars which are used to provide tender care for our crippled children, our blind and our deaf, our dumb, our pitiful, aged and infirm, to build highways, hospitals and school, then certainly I am in favor of it.

This is my stand. I will not retreat from it. I will not compromise.
Address to legislature by a Mississippi senator in 1958.

Substance abuse, or chemical dependency, has been proclaimed the third most important health problem in our country by the Surgeon General, and yet our attitudes as a society exhibit much ambivalence toward alcohol and drugs.

Over 50 percent of all traffic fatalities are alcohol-related. One third of suicides are committed by alcoholics. Alcoholics are ten times more likely to die from fires than nonalcoholics and five to thirteen times more likely to die from falls. Chronic brain injury caused by alcohol is second only to Alzheimer's disease as a known cause of mental deterioration in adults. Fetal alcohol syndrome is the third leading cause of birth defects with mental retardation—and the only preventable one. Twenty to 50 percent of admissions to general hospitals are for alcohol-related problems. Fifty-four percent of jail inmates convicted of violent crimes were drinking before they committed the offense. Drinking is estimated to be involved in 50 percent of spouse abuse and 38 percent of child abuse. One out of three American adults say that alcohol abuse has brought trouble to his or her family. Children of alcoholics have a four times greater risk of developing alcoholism than children of nonalcoholics and are 50 percent more likely to marry an alcoholic person.

At least 500,000 Americans are addicted to heroin; at least 1 million abuse tranquilizers daily; 53 million have used marijuana, and up to 20 million have tried cocaine or crack. In Baltimore during an eleven-year period, 231 heroin addicts committed 500,000 crimes. Several years ago the Justice Department found that heroin addicts alone committed 20 percent of all property crimes. Between 1976 and 1986 there was a fifteenfold increase in emergency-room visits attributed to cocaine use, cocaine-related deaths (more than 5 per 1,000 deaths), and in admissions to cocaine-treatment programs. By 1986 almost 15 percent of the United States population had tried cocaine. A Gallup campus poll in 1986 found that more than half of the 516 college students interviewed had tried marijuana. Three quarters of the students identified marijuana as the drug they used most often.

Chemical dependency is one of three top killer diseases and the number one cause of death among fifteen- to twenty-four-year-olds. When we add nicotine, drug abuse becomes the number one cause of death in our society.

In 1987, $120 billion was the cost to the nation of alcohol abuse, and yet the congressional research appropriation for alcohol abuse was less than $1 million. The economic cost to the nation of drug abuse in 1987 was $63 billion, and congressional research appropriations were $101,500. Yet when we compare the cost to the nation of cardiovascular disease ($80 billion) or cancer ($70 billion), we find that the congressional research appropriations are much more equitable (cardiovascular disease—$.75 billion, cancer—$1 billion).

Alcoholism occurs in one out of ten people who drink alcohol. The average alcoholic is in his or her midforties with a responsible job and family. Only 5 percent of alcoholics are Skid Row bums.

Drugs of abuse are chemical substances that alter mood, perception, or consciousness. The drugs of abuse can be divided into classes: depressants (including alcohol), stimulants, narcotics, hallucinogens, and cannabis. Each class will be discussed individually, emphasizing effects on the body and the mind. It is to be understood that while the effects of each class can be generalized, there is marked individual variation as to the expression of these effects. The exact amount of frequency of drug required to produce certain effects is variable for each individual.

DEPENDENCY SUBSTANCES

Depressants

The depressants include tranquilizers, sleeping pills, and alcohol; they are the most commonly abused legal drugs. The common effects of these drugs are relaxation, euphoria, somnolence, and in higher doses slurred speech, disorientation, and drunken behavior. Overdose causes shallow respiration, cold and clammy skin, dilated pupils, weak and rapid pulse, and possible death. When these drugs are used regularly and stopped suddenly, a withdrawal syndrome may occur, including anxiety, difficulty sleeping, tremors, confusion, convulsions, and possible death. Table 3 lists the most commonly used depressants. All of the depressants affect the brain. Alcohol affects not only the brain but almost every organ system. The organ system affected varies from individual to individual, depending on many factors including genetic predisposition. However, the majority of people who drink heavily will have some of the mentioned physical consequences.

TABLE 2 COMMONLY USED DEPRESSANTS

Valium	Miltown
Librium	Butisol
Ativan	Dalmane
Xanax	Restoril
Centrax	Halcion
Tranxene	Seconal
Fiorinal	Nembutal
Phrenilin	

Alcohol first causes euphoria by depressing the inhibitory center of the brain, resulting in a feeling of relaxation. As the level of alcohol increases in the brain, judgment is impaired, speech becomes slurred. There is difficulty with coordination, producing the characteristic drunken gait. There may be sudden changes in mood, producing inappropriate laughter or crying. Eventually, as the level increases, the person goes into a stupor, and if the blood-alcohol level is high enough, respiratory depression occurs and death ensues.

The well-known hangover is withdrawal from a large alcohol dose and is characterized by anxiety, tremors, difficulty sleeping, nausea, and headache. More serious withdrawal or major withdrawal symptoms include fever, high blood pressure, rapid pulse, sweating, hallucinations, delusions, and seizures and is more commonly called DTs or delirium tremens. Approximately 15 percent of people in DTs will die. The withdrawal effects of the other depressant drugs are very similar to alcohol, but occur at different times. Whereas the minor withdrawal symptoms of alcohol occur twelve to twenty-four hours after the last drink and the major symptoms occur forty-eight to seventy-two hours after the last drink, the benzodiazepams (Valium, Librium, Xanax, and many others) often produce a withdrawal that starts about seven to ten days after the last dose and lasts sometimes for weeks or months. The treatment of the withdrawal symptoms includes giving large doses of another depressant drug and decreasing the dosage of the drug until the symptoms have completely abated. All depressant drugs are then discontinued. Long-term use of depressant drugs is contraindicated and has actually been associated with addiction or relapse.

Besides affecting the brain, the most common medical complications of alcohol abuse or dependence involve the gastrointestinal system. Alcohol acts as an irritant, and excessive quantities often cause inflammation of the esophagus and stomach, produce vomiting, abdominal pain and sometimes vomiting blood. It produces diarrhea and poor absorption of nutrients. There is an increased incidence of cancer of the esophagus with heavy alcohol and cigarette consumption. Pancreatitis (inflammation of the pancreas) is associated with heavy alcohol use and is characterized by abdominal pain boring through to the back, and vomiting. It is diagnosed by characteristic abnormalities found in the bloodstream (i.e., elevated amylase). As alcohol continues to have an effect on the pancreas, it can cause chronic pancreatitis, resulting in diabetes and severe malnutrition, often leading to death.

Alcohol is detoxified in the liver and initially causes an accumulation of fat in that organ, resulting in a large liver and characteristically abnormal laboratory tests. Once drinking has stopped, the fat disappears, the liver becomes normal in size, and the laboratory tests return to normal. Alcoholic hepatitis is a result of direct injury to the liver cell and is a much more serious condition, causing fever, jaundice, (yellow skin), nausea, and lethargy. In contrast to the alcoholic fatty liver, recovery from alcoholic hepatitis is not as predictable. When alcohol is stopped completely, 80 percent of patients improve or recover, but 20 percent progress to serious disease. If alcohol use is continued, 50–80 percent progress to cirrhosis and 30–50 percent continue as alcoholic hepatitis. The most serious result of alcohol's effect on the liver is cirrhosis, in which the normal liver cells are replaced by scar tissue.

The liver has many functions in the body, and the more of cells are replaced by scar tissue, the more abnormal the liver function becomes and the sicker the person. A common function of the liver is manufacturing body proteins, some of which help with immunity from infections, with blood clotting, with building body cells, and with maintaining proper amounts of fluid in the vascular system. The liver also clears bilirubin from the blood, secreting it into the gallbladder, which later helps with digestion. The liver processes ammonia, which is a metabolic end product or toxin produced by cell metabolism. When these normal functions of the liver are interrupted, the ammonia builds up, often causing coma and death. In addition, infections occur; the blood does not clot normally; bilirubin accumulates in the blood, producing jaundice, and the vascular system is unable to hold sufficient fluid, so swelling develops, mostly in the legs and abdomen. Large amounts of scar tissue in the liver also produce obstruction to the flow of blood through the veins, which normally courses through the liver, and this in turn results in the ballooning of the vein that drains the spleen. An enlarged, congested spleen can rupture and cause death, or the ballooning veins themselves may rupture, causing a possibly fatal hemorrhage. Once alcoholic cirrhosis is diagnosed, if alcohol consumption is stopped, there is a 64 percent chance of survival at the end of five years. If alcohol consumption continues, there is a 40 percent chance of survival at the end of five years.

Heavy consumption of alcohol also affects the immune system. There is a decrease in the manufacture of proteins by the liver and the number of white cells, which normally help with resistance to bacteria. The latter is a result of alcohol's effect on bone marrow, the blood-forming organ.

Alcohol affects the cardiovascular system most commonly by producing hypertension. When alcohol consumption is stopped, the blood pressure often goes down to normal. Alcohol also directly affects the heart by causing a condition called cardiomyopathy. The heart muscle stretches and becomes less efficient, so that the heart is enlarged and is unable to pump the blood normally. This causes congestive heart failure, in which the blood backs up in the lungs and in the rest of the body, causing shortness of breath and swelling. Alcohol can cause an irregular heartbeat often referred to as the "holiday heart," because this problem occurs most frequently during holiday times, when there is heavy alcohol consumption.

Alcohol affects the glandular system of the body, primarily in the area of sexual functioning. Male alcoholics often have a decreased libido, which may progress to impotence caused both by alcohol's effects on sexual hormone production by the brain and by its direct effect on the testicles. Usually the impotence is reversible if the testicles are normal size. If they are small, it is often irreversible, even when alcohol is discontinued. Alcohol may also cause enlarged breasts in men, because of an inability of the liver to metabolize normally circulating female hormones (estrogen). Excessive alcohol intake in women often leads to irregular or excessive menses, sometimes requiring gynecologic surgical procedures (i.e., D & Cs and hysterectomies). There is also an increased incidence of premenstrual syndrome in women who drink alcohol excessively.

Excessive alcohol intake during pregnancy often affects the fetus. Alcohol crosses the placenta freely, so that as the mother is drinking, so is the baby. The effects on the baby depend on the trimester of pregnancy in which the heavy drinking occurs. During the first trimester (the first three months), the major organs and structures of the body are being formed, so that during this period, there are more likely to be abnormalities of the internal organs, the brain, the face, and the heart. During the second three months, there is an increased risk of miscarriage. During the third three months, there is decreased fetal growth, which produces a small, lightweight baby. Even moderate drinking during pregnancy has been shown to produce decreased birth weight. The fetal alcohol syndrome, which is the most severe manifestation of fetal abnormalities, may produce a baby with shorter length than average, with less weight than average and a smaller head, with characteristically abnormal facial appearance, and with mental retardation. In July 1981, the surgeon general advised women who were pregnant or considering becoming pregnant not to drink alcoholic beverages at all.

Alcohol affects the nervous system in many ways. Excessive alcohol intake over many years can produce permanent brain damage, resulting in inappropriate judgment, diminished memory, confusion, and rigidity of thinking. Alcohol also affects the peripheral nerves, producing symptoms of burning and numbness of the feet and difficulty walking. Many of the effects on the nervous system are thought to be due also to deficiency of the B vitamins. At times these symptoms can be reversed with high doses of B vitamins and abstinence from alcohol. At times, they may be irreversible.

Cannabis

Cannabis is the class of drugs that includes marijuana and hashish, the resin of the marijuana plant. Marijuana, the leaf, is the most commonly abused illegal drug and is often referred to as a gateway drug, in that once a person has tried marijuana, he has gained access into the illegal drug scene and is more likely to continue on to other illegal drugs such as cocaine and heroin. The immediate effects of smoking marijuana, the most common form

Substance Abuse 143

of intake, include increased heart rate, red eyes, dry mouth, mild euphoria, changes in perception, heightened appreciation of sounds and colors, apparent slowdown in passage of time, disturbance of short-term memory, impairment of coordination. Long-term effects (frequent heavy usage over several months to years) include psychological dependency, a decreased motivation, interference with learning, and the amotivational syndrome in which a person stops attending school or stops working, and chooses instead to use the drug. There is also some evidence that marijuana causes bronchitis, lung cancer, decreased immune response, and may make asthma or angina pectoris worse. Marijuana is not physically addicting and does not have a withdrawal syndrome.

Hallucinogens

Hallucinogens include LSD, mescaline, peyote, and phencyclidine or PCP and some type of designer drugs, which are synthetic drugs made to resemble other psychoactive drugs. These drugs are most usually taken in pill form by mouth. PCP can be smoked or injected by vein. These drugs change perception by causing hallucinations and poor perception of time and distance. Longer, more increased use and heavy dosage may produce psychosis (complete separation from reality) and possible death. There is no withdrawal syndrome from these drugs, but they may produce psychological dependence.

Stimulants

Stimulant drugs include cocaine, amphetamines or speed, and diet pills (Preludin and Tenuate). Caffeine and nicotine are also in this class. The most commonly abused illegal drug in this class is cocaine, and its use has increased markedly over the last few years. It is snorted (inhaled and absorbed through the mucous membranes of the nose), smoked, or injected directly into the bloodstream. It is more rapidly addicting when it is smoked or injected because it gets to the brain faster. Crack is a form of cocaine that is smoked. Cocaine is a very addicting drug, and experiments on rats have found that when they become dependent on it, they prefer cocaine over food, sex, or water and will die from malnutrition. The other stimulants are usually taken by mouth or injected. The immediate effects of cocaine and the other stimulants include increased energy, euphoria, decreased hunger, elevated blood pressure, and pulse. The effects last about thirty minutes and then a rather severe lethargy and depression may occur. Deaths can occur immediately from the effects of cocaine or the stimulants by respiratory depression, seizures, heart attacks, or strokes. Stimulants act as constrictors of the arteries and decrease the blood supply to the organ affected. When a stroke is caused, it indicates that the blood supply to the brain has been cut off. When a heart attack occurs, the blood supply to the heart is severely limited. Withdrawal from stimulants causes depression and lethargy, and although it is usually not directly life threatening, suicide may be a real risk.

Narcotics

"Narcotics" includes heroin, obtained illegally, but also many drugs commonly used in medicine for relief of pain. (See Table 4). The narcotics produce euphoria, relieve pain, and tend to cause the pupils to constrict and the gastrointestinal system to slow down. Overdoses of narcotics cause slow and shallow breathing, eventually resulting in respiratory depression and death. Withdrawal symptoms from narcotics include watery eyes, runny nose, yawning, loss of appetite, irritability, tremors, panic, chills, sweating, cramps, and nausea. Though the withdrawal symptoms may be severe, and very uncomfortable, they are not life threatening and do not produce death as withdrawal symptoms from the depressants have been known to do.

TABLE 3: COMMONLY USED NARCOTICS

Darvocet N	Demerol
Darvon	Stadol
Dilaudid	Nubain
Tylox	Percodan
Codeine	Percocet
Tylenol #2, #3, #4	Vicodin
(Tylenol-codeine combinations)	

Diagnosis of Addiction

Almost any drug can be injected IV, but heroin or cocaine are most commonly used in this fashion. Complications resulting from intravenous drug use often have little or no bearing on the actual drug injected but have to do with the injection process itself. Often the drug-dependent person will share needles with other drug-dependent people and thus risk infection. Infections may be bacterial, producing septicemia or blood poisoning, local abscesses, or endocarditis (infections of the heart valve) or they may be viral (most commonly hepatitis B or AIDS). There also can be complications from injecting toxic substances that are used to cut the drug, and these can result in abnormalities of the lungs and brain and severe allergic reactions.

ADDICTION. ABUSE, AND DEPENDENCE

Addiction to any substance has been defined by David Smith, M.D., of the Haight-Ashbury Clinic in San Francisco, as "compulsion, loss of control and continued use in spite of adverse consequences." The adverse consequences are most likely marital or family problems, job problems, legal problems, health problems, or financial problems.

A definition of terms commonly used may clarify a rather complex concept. *Drug abuse* implies excessive use of a drug on one or more occasions, which caused harm to the individual or to others. *Drug dependence* occurs when a person cannot function normally without the repeated use of the drug, and the person has severe physical and psychological disturbances when the drug is withdrawn. Not all the drugs of abuse produce dependence. For example, the hallucinogens (LSD and marijuana) can be abused and yet do not produce a withdrawal reaction when discontinued. Addiction may include drug abuse and/or drug dependence, but its hallmark is compulsion and loss of control. Drug abuse and drug dependence may exist without addiction; for example, one episode of a hangover from alcohol without subsequent episodes or one episode of a heavy crack smoking with subsequent complete abstinence from cocaine do not constitute addiction. Drug dependence may occur in any person who is on a prolonged course of narcotics under medical supervision for severe pain. The characteristic physical withdrawal symptoms will occur, but subsequently the person who is not addicted will not seek out the narcotic.

Addiction itself is a well-recognized disease entity. Alcoholism was proclaimed a disease by the American Medical Association in 1956. Chemical dependency was recognized as a disease by the American Medical Association in 1987. A disease has been defined as "a definite morbid process having a characteristic train of symptoms. It may affect the whole body or any of its parts and its etiology, pathology, and prognosis may be known or unknown." Chemical dependency has symptoms that can be described, the course of the illness is predictable and progressive, and the disease is primary, meaning that it is not just a symptom of some underlying disorder. It is permanent. Once addicted, a person cannot safely return to the use of potentially addicting drugs. If left untreated, it often results in premature death.

The disease of addition can be divided into early, middle, and late stages.

Early stage Early stage symptoms are listed in Table 4 below.

TABLE 4: EARLY STAGE SYMPTOMS OF ADDICTION

Preoccupation	Solitary drinking
Increased tolerance for alcohol	Blackouts
Rapid intake	Protection for supply
Use of alcohol as medicine	Nonpremeditated

Preoccupation occurs when the person affected thinks or talks about drinking or using his drug when he should be concerned with other matters. Focusing on the experience of "getting high" is the initial and continuing hallmark of any kind of drug addiction. *Increased tolerance* indicates that it takes more and more of the drug or alcohol to produce the desired effect. The early-stage alcoholic is able to drink much more than the normal drinker before he becomes intoxicated. *Rapid intake* indicates that a person takes the drug or alcohol in such a manner that it will act quickly upon him. The alcoholic often orders a double shot and may gulp drinks. He also may take a drink before going to a party. *Use as medicine* occurs when a person uses his drug of choice at night to help him get to sleep or will use it when he feels ill, either physically or emotionally. If he feels unusually anxious or depressed he may use his drink or drug of choice. *Using alone* is often a hallmark of early addiction. The alcoholic will often drink at home when no one else is drinking or will stop in a bar and drink by himself. Drinking alone is not social drinking. *Blackout* is an experience of amnesia. Sometimes, on the morning after a drinking bout, the alcoholic has difficulty recalling some of the events of the previous evening. Memory for these particular events never come back. *Protecting the supply* is the tendency of the alcoholic to hide alcohol or drug of choice, or put it in inappropriate places like the desk at the office or in the car to assure that there is always some on hand. *Unpremeditated use* describes the tendency of the alcoholic or drug addict to use or drink more than intended or to use or drink when he had previously decided not to. *Loss of control* is the hallmark of any kind of drug addiction. Once the person starts using his drug of choice or alcohol, he is unable to control the amount and will often continue to use it until he is ill or unconscious. This statement may be misleading in that many an alcoholic or addict may appear to have control on occasions but will subsequently lose it repeatedly.

Middle stage: The middle stage of chemical dependency is characterized by progressive loss of control of drug or alcohol use. There is considerable remorse and guilt. There may be periods of abstinence followed by binges. Alibis and excuses may be used too. Family, friends, and coworkers may begin to show some concern. There may be financial problems and the eye-opener or the drink upon awakening may be necessary to function.

Late stage: The late stage is characterized by losses. Severe withdrawal symptoms (when alcohol is involved) occurs. The tolerance, which initially was increased, may start decreasing, and it takes less and less of the alcohol or drug to produce the same effect. There tends to be moral and ethical deterioration, increasing medical problems and repeated hospital visits, loss of family, friends, and job. There may be incarcerations or permanent brain damage. The end stage of dependence on drugs or alcohol, if left untreated, is death.

CAUSE OF ADDICTION

Addiction is thought to have complex causes. Research is showing that there is a large genetic component to this disease. Children born to alcoholic parents, but raised by nonalcoholic parents, are more likely to become alcoholic than the reverse—that is children of nonalcoholic parents raised by alcoholic parents. Indeed, sons of alcoholics are four times more likely to contract the disease of alcoholism than sons of nonalcoholics. Identical-twin studies have also indicated that when one twin is alcoholic, the other twin is much more likely to have the disease than a nonidentical twin. Animal research has indicated that mice can be bred to become alcoholic. Recent studies on sons of alcoholic fathers have shown differences in brain waves (EEGs) and initial increase in tolerance to alcohol compared to children of nonalcoholics (1).

Chemicals may play a part. It has been discovered that many chemicals that function as neurotransmitters are present within the brain. These include dopamine, serotonin, norepinephrine, and endorphins (the "feel good" chemicals). It is thought that addiction may be due to a disorder in the complex interactions of these chemicals, and by using his drug, whatever it is, the affected person may be trying to change the chemical reactions of the brain. There is considerable individual variability as to which drug is preferred, and this individual preference may relate to individual differences of interrelationships of the various chemicals (2). Research continues on this complicated subject.

Once a person is addicted to one drug (or to alcohol), he is more likely to become addicted to another. Increasingly, people are found to be addicted to several drugs of abuse rather than to a single one. When alcoholics are given tranquilizers, they may become addicted to both alcohol and to the tranquilizer. Heroin addicts treated successfully for heroin addiction become alcoholic at least 50 percent of the time. Cocaine addicts have a strong family history of alcoholism. Addiction appears to be the feeling of intoxication, the high produced by the drug, and if the addict is unable to obtain his drug of choice, he will use another.

TREATMENT

Once a patient has been diagnosed for alcoholism or chemical dependency, he should be started on a treatment program. However, before that can take place, the patient probably has to go through the stage called denial. Denial is defined as the inability of a person to see the seriousness of his or her problem. But concerned family, friends, and professionals can help to break through this denial by a process called the intervention. The intervention process was originated by Vern Johnson and is well described in his book, *I'll Quit Tomorrow* (3).

The concerned group meets with the chemically dependent person, preferably at a time when he is not under the influence of the drug or alcohol. The goal of this meeting is to confront him with his behavior while under the influence and show what effect this behavior had on others, in particular the people at the meeting. It is very important that this be done in nonjudgmental fashion. During a typical intervention, the wife of an alcoholic may list events in their married life that have been upsetting to her: embarrassing her at a party because of drunken behavior, forgetting to pick up children when asked to, staying out all night on several occasions, being verbally—possibly even physically—abusive at times, and so on. Each participant in the intervention process proceeds to describe—being nonjudgmental, caring, but realistic—drug-related actions of the patient and how they have affected him, the speaker. Each participant, while expressing his feelings with warmth and consideration, nevertheless presents reality without sparing the patient's feelings. When people who are close to the affected person have shared their perceptions with such honesty, he will often realize the effect his disease has had on others—and himself—and will then become receptive to receiving treatment.

Before the intervention has taken place, a treatment plan will already have been planned, and if the intervention is successful, the patient is taken directly to a treatment program. The intervention process is a very delicate but powerful tool, and should be directed by a trained chemical-dependency counselor or physician with a knowledge of addictions. Appropriate treatment facilities can be recommended by them, too.

Treatment of chemical dependency is a fourfold process: physical, emotional, mental, and spiritual. It must start with the physical component. The patient must be safely detoxified, if necessary, and any medical problems

Substance Abuse

he has need to be addressed before further treatment can be undertaken. For some individuals, appropriately screened, detoxification may be done on an outpatient basis if closely monitored by well-trained professionals. Other patients must be admitted to the hospital for closer observation, especially when there is danger of DTs or seizures.

Once the patient is physically stabilized, the emotional aspects of his disease can be treated. Most people with addictive diseases have had difficulty recognizing and expressing normal human emotions. Anger and fear are normal emotions shared by all human beings, but are extremely threatening to those with addictions, so for years before treatment, they have covered up those emotions with their drugs. What the addicted person most commonly feels is numbness; other feelings, which begin to surface during the early recovery period, seem very powerful and frightening. Group therapy is extremely effective in helping the chemically dependent patient recognize and handle these normal feelings.

Group therapy is also helpful in treating the mental aspects of this disease. Most people with active addictions tend to be very rigid in their thought processes and may have poor judgment. Successful recovery from this disease necessitates an ever-increasing flexibility in thinking and a more accepting attitude toward life and others.

The spiritual component of the disease is important for the success of long-term recovery. Spirituality can be defined as knowing who one is and who one is not. It can best he summed up in the serenity prayer which is recited at every Alcoholics Anonymous meeting: "God grant me the serenity to accept the things I cannot change, the courage to change the things I can, and the wisdom to know the difference." The person who begins to grow spiritually begins to learn to love and accept himself as he is, to love and accept others as they are, and to love and accept life as it is. This is a lifetime journey.

This treatment for chemical dependency may take place in an inpatient rehabilitation unit or in an outpatient program or by heavily concentrated attendance at meetings of Alcoholics Anonymous and/or Narcotics Anonymous. Effective treatment is a bridge between active addictive behavior and a recovery-oriented life-style. It is based on active participation in a Twelve Step Program (see below). Successful recovery from chemical dependency almost always parallels growth and active participation in the Twelve Step Program.

THE TWELVE STEPS OF ALCOHOLIC ANONYMOUS
(With Modifications for Narcotics Anonymous and Alanon)

1. We admitted we were powerless over alcohol/addiction—that our lives had become unmanageable.

2. Came to believe that a Power greater than ourselves could restore us to sanity.
3. Made a decision to turn our will and our lives over to the care of God *as we understood him.*
4. Made a searching and fearless moral inventory of ourselves.
5. Admitted to God, to ourselves, and to another human being the exact nature of our wrongs.
6. Were entirely ready to have God remove all these defects of character.
7. Humbly asked Him to remove our shortcomings.
8. Made a list of all persons we had harmed and became willing to make amends to them all.
9. Made direct amends to such people wherever possible, except when to do so would injure them or others.
10. Continued to take personal inventory, and when we were wrong, promptly admitted it.
11. Sought through prayer and meditation to improve our conscious contact with God *as we understood him,* praying only for knowledge of His will for us and the power to carry that out.
12. Having had a spiritual awakening as the results of these steps, we tried to carry this message to alcoholics, addicts, and others, and to practice these principles in all our affairs.

Effective treatment programs, both inpatient and outpatient, have an aftercare component, meaning regular attendance at structured meetings run by these programs for as much as a year to two years after the initial treatment. The cooperation of the patient's family and/or close friends plays a vital role in aftercare; they receive education about the disease of chemical dependency and especially about the family illness and thus learn the most appropriate ways to support the patient's recovery. The success of the patient has been found to depend largely on the strength of these aftercare programs.

THE FAMILY ILLNESS OF CHEMICAL DEPENDENCY

The disease of chemical dependency is very subtle in the beginning and as it progresses, the family, close friends, and even coworkers of the patient often become part of the disease—unwillingly involved in his continuing addiction. As they attempt to make adjustments to the chemically dependent person's progressive disease, they develop behavior and/or emotional problems of their own. Family members often *encourage* the drug seeking or drinking behavior of the alcoholic/addict without realizing it.

We call such people enablers—individuals who react to a chemically dependent person by shielding him from the harmful consequences of his disease. The enabler helps the chemically dependent person delude himself that using the drug or drinking is not the problem. A wife, for example, calls her husband's employer to tell him that John (actually hungover) can't come to work because he has the flu. Other family members—often, tragically, children—may take on the responsibilities of the home when the drug-addicted or alcoholic mother is unable to function. A parent may repeatedly bail his drug-addicted adolescent out of jail excusing the youngster's behavior as "teenage acting out" and preventing him or her from experiencing the full impact of dependency. Many family members are embarrassed about the alcoholic or drug-addicted behavior of other members and hide this from outsiders, further delaying the diagnosis of the illness.

After a while, the family, friends, and close coworkers tend to let their response to the sick behavior become the center of their lives. Many times they do this out of fear, and many times they do this out of misplaced kindness, thinking they are being helpful, supportive, and loving. Any family member or friend who does for the chemically dependent person what that person should be doing for himself is enabling.

Of course, if the wife doesn't cover up for her husband, he may actually lose his job, but it may become necessary for him to lose his job anyway—in order to get real help for his problem. As long as the problem is being covered up, it will never be confronted directly. Enablers often act out of soft-heartedness and sympathy, but more of the time this backfires. Sometimes enablers try to control the drug use or alcohol by getting rid of the substance—but more is always available. Or the enabler may try to make the environment more pleasing to the chemically dependent person by changing his behavior. An example of this may be a wife who begins to clean her house, obsessively and compulsively, cook gourmet meals, keep the children quiet—all in an effort to lessen stress and decrease the need for her husband to drink. What she doesn't realize is that stress is not the cause of the drinking. Many times, close family members—even children—feel that the drinking or drugging behavior of the affected person is their fault. This also is not true. The drinking is a disease and not under their control.

The thrust of treatment for the family members is education. They must learn about the disease of chemical dependency and how to let go of responsibility for the chemically dependent person's drinking or drug use and subsequent behavior. The family members are introduced to Alanon, a Twelve Step Program for families and friends of alcoholics, and Alateen, a Twelve Step Program for teenage children of alcoholics. There is also Naranon for families of narcotic addicts.

Earlier in this chapter, it was mentioned that children of alcoholics were

50 percent more likely to marry an alcoholic than children of nonalcoholics. In family treatment, the spouse of the chemically dependent person begins to understand the effect that chemically dependency has had on his or her life, even before the present marriage relationship, and many times it is necessary for family members to obtain more counseling. Again their recovery is largely dependent on continuation and active participation in the Twelve Step Program of Alanon or Naranon.

Increasingly dependency experts are learning to recognize the characteristics of adult children of alcoholics. These are people who grew up in a home, in which one or both parents was an alcoholic or a drug addict. Characteristics of such adult children include the following: (1) isolation and fear of people and authority figures; (2) overwhelming need for approval from others; (3) fear of angry people and any personal criticism; (4) increased tendency to become alcoholic or chemically dependent themselves or to marry dependents; (5) a tendency to live life from the viewpoint of a victim; (6) an overdeveloped sense of responsibility; (7) guilt feelings when standing up for their own rights; (8) addiction to excitement; (9) difficulty recognizing and expressing feelings; (10) low sense of self-esteem; (11) overwhelming dependence on relationships and fear of abandonment.

Persons suffering from the above characteristics can receive help from individual counseling or by participating in Alanon, which now has a branch called Adult Children of Alcoholics, a group which meets under a Twelve Step Program.

This chapter has been limited to the discussion of abuse of drugs and alcohol, but a more thorough discussion would include food, sex, relationships, gambling, power, money, work, etc. Any addiction to any of these substances or conditions or behaviors implies that a person is seeking from outside sources (a substance, another person, an activity), a feeling which in a healthier person would arrive from within. All people with addictions have low self-esteem and depend on substances, other people, or activities to bolster that esteem. Recovery from any addiction necessitates continual growth and self-acceptance, acceptance of others, and acceptance of life.

7

NUTRITION
Patricia Sumko-Imhof, R.D.

Nutrition is a science, a new science, continuing to evolve. Because eating habits and styles are so personal—raising strong emotions established early in life—the truth about food and nutrition is frequently distorted.

Bookstores are full of self-help books: nutrition and weight-loss; nutrition and longevity; nutrition and disease prevention; nutrition and exercise; nutrition and every-period-of-the-life-cycle. Probably as many nutrition books are based on fiction as are based on fact, and many others mix both together. It is a characteristic of human nature to believe that there can be simple solutions to everything, such as taking a nutrient supplement or powder to improve health. This, coupled with the current demand for nutrition information, has created a mass of nutrition *mis*information. The objective of this chapter is to present the facts, identify what aspects of nutrition are currently under investigation, and put food and healthful eating into perspective.

Simply defined, nutrition is the food we eat and how our bodies use it for growth and maintaining health. A body's need for nutrients varies during the life cycle. Sex, age, size, hereditary factors, and one's health and the presence of disease or metabolic stress all play a part. The fifty-plus nutrients required by the body on an everyday basis are available in a wide variety of foods. No one food or food group has them all. The wider the variety of foods chosen, especially fruits, vegetables, and grains, the greater the nutritional value and balance of the overall diet. The variety factor helps to ensure the body of getting the necessary nutrients without excesses. It also helps to prevent overingestion of any one preservative, herbicide, pesticide, or questionable additive. Additionally, many nutrients work together. So a wide variety of foods will provide the right mix of nutrients for optimal function, besides making meals more interesting and enjoyable.

The adage "the key to life is moderation" couldn't be more true for nutrition. One of the reasons vitamin supplements are so misused is because of the conviction that, if a little bit is good, then ten times more is ten times better. Another common nutrition mistake is in thinking that some foods are "bad" or "fattening" whereas others are "good" or "reducing." If the overall diet is varied and well-balanced, a piece of chocolate cake has little effect on the individual's overall nutritional status. On the other hand, if breakfast is skipped, the midmorning snack consists of coffee with cream and a doughnut, lunch is from a vending machine, and supper is a typical fast-food meal, a piece of fruit before bed will not correct a day's worth of unwise food choices. There are choices between skim milk and whole milk, a bran muffin and a frosted sweet roll, a 4-ounce steak and a 10-ounce steak, margarine and butter, cantaloupe with fresh blueberries and apple pie a la mode, sorbet and gourmet ice cream, steamed asparagus and deep-fried cauliflower, a baked potato and french fries. How much and how often are choices too. Each of us is personally responsible to ourselves for the food choices we make everyday, every meal, every snack.

UNDERSTANDING THE BASICS

To simplify a complex subject, nutrients are divided into six major categories: proteins, fats, carbohydrates, vitamins, minerals, and water (1). Most foods are a combination of two or more of the major nutrients. Whole milk, for example, contains all six. Bread is a combination of predominantly carbohydrate, some protein, vitamins, minerals, and very little water or fat. Fats like margarine and butter are just that—about 99 percent fat by weight; butter contains vitamin A naturally whereas margarine is fortified with vitamin A. The reduced-calorie margarines have water added. Fruits have a very high water content, which is why they are naturally low in calories. They also contain a considerable amount of vitamins and minerals. A brief description of each category follows.

Proteins

Proteins are molecules composed of amino acids, which are made of common elements including carbon, hydrogen, oxygen, nitrogen, and sometimes sulfur. Amino acids are the building blocks of proteins, which determine their multiple functions. Protein exists in the structure of all living organisms. It forms the bone, muscle, skin, brain, red blood cells, and all the other organs and tissues of the human body. Proteins also carry out many functions in the body. As enzymes, they control chemical reactions. As hormones, they act as messengers regulating various body processes. As antibodies, they function as part of the immune system—able to recognize and destroy foreign substances. Proteins also act as carriers to transport various molecules across cell membranes or in the blood. One protein, hemoglobin, transports oxygen from the lungs to the cells. Albumin, a protein in the blood, carries the minerals calcium and zinc throughout the body.

There are over twenty different amino acids. Eight of these amino acids are classified as essential, meaning the body is unable to produce them, and we must obtain them from the food we eat. All of the other amino acids can be produced by the body when the eight essentials are consumed daily. After a meal, the digestive process will begin, and the protein foods consumed will be broken down into their individual amino acids. All the essential amino acids must be present in adequate amounts for the synthesis of a new protein to take place. Foods that contain all the essential amino acids, in the correct proportions, are considered "complete" proteins. Only foods of animal origin, like meat and milk, are complete. Eggs, for all the bad press they have received for their cholesterol content, are actually classified as the perfect protein. This is because the egg's amino-acid composition has "high biological value"—meaning it provides all the essential amino acids in the correct proportions necessary for the body to use. All other protein foods are compared to the egg and assigned a number less than 100 (the egg is 100) in relationship to the amino-acid composition. Foods of plant origin like beans, bread, rice, and vegetables also contain protein but are considered "incomplete," because they are missing one or more of the essential amino acids. When an incomplete protein food like legumes (dried beans, peas, lentils)—which are low in the amino acids methionine and cystine but high in lysine—are combined with corn—which is low in lysine but adequate in methionine and cystine—a complete protein is the result. Serving cornbread with a meatless chili or Mexican tostadas with corn tortillas and beans results in a complete protein formed from two incomplete proteins. The fundamental structure of a vegetarian diet is based on protein complementation.

The best food sources of protein are eggs, fish and seafood, poultry, beef, pork, lamb, veal, milk, yogurt, and cheese. However, it is possible to consume an adequate amount and quality of protein without eating meat. Many nutrition experts are encouraging people to reduce their intake of animal proteins and increase the amount of plant proteins in their diet. This is not to say a vegetarian style of eating is appropriate for everyone, and indeed a strict vegan type of vegetarianism is actually quite dangerous. But because of the affluence and abundance which exist in the United States, many Americans consume one and a half to two times more protein than they need.

An obvious question is how much protein is enough on a daily basis? Well, it depends. A newborn infant, who will triple his birth weight by age one, is building new cells at a very fast rate. Protein needs are based on actual weight for infants and ideal body weight for height, as a person ages. So the infant needs about 2.2 grams (g) of protein per kilogram (kg) to meet the demands of growth, where the healthy adult needs only .8 g/kg of ideal body weight for maintenance and repair purposes. For example, a thirty-year-old, 5 foot 7 inch woman, who is at her ideal body weight of 135 pounds, needs 62 g of protein per day to meet her protein needs. Two 8-ounce glasses of skim milk and 7 ounces of lean meat, fish, or poultry (cooked weight) alone will provide all the protein this woman needs. A man's need for protein is greater, proportional to his greater body weight.

Protein needs are greater during the growth phases of life cycle, pregnancy, and lactation, then level off for the healthy adult. Periods of stress such as major surgery will increase protein needs. Or if an individual suffers a major injury like third-degree burns over a high percentage of the body, protein requirements will increase to that of the newborn, to facilitate the healing process and build new cells. Additional protein beyond what the body needs serves no additional benefit. If anything, it is a burden to the body, specifically the kidneys. Extra protein may be used for energy purposes. However, it is not an efficient fuel, and it's quite an expensive fuel source at that.

Fats

The more technical term for fat is "lipid." Lipids are defined as a class of biomolecules that are insoluble in water. Obvious examples of dietary fat are butter, margarine, and oils. Less obvious examples of "invisible fats" include cheese, whole milk, pastries, red meats, and some types of crackers. Lipids serve a number of important functions in the body, acting as essential constituents in the structure of membranes, as a concentrated source of energy, and as an insulator and protective padding of internal organs; they also perform such specialized functions as carrying the fat-soluble vitamins and comprising a portion of some hormones (1).

Lipids are classified into a number of subcategories, but for practical purposes, only fatty acids and cholesterol will be considered here. The term "cholesterol" is probably the most familiar. "Saturated fats," "polyunsaturated oils," and "hydrogenated margarines" are becoming common household words. Recently a few newcomers like "monounsaturated fats," "Omega-3 fatty acids," and "canola oil" have been added. In spite of the efforts of scientists, nutritionists, physicians, and such organizations as the American Heart Association, most people remain confused about the relationship of fats in the diet to the development of heart disease. Considering the complexity of the problem and decades of controversial research, it's no wonder fats are so misunderstood.

Like proteins, fats are comprised of common elements—carbon, hydrogen, and oxygen. The chemical structure and certain characteristics of the fat determine whether it is a saturated or unsaturated fatty acid. In simple terms, a fat is saturated when there is a hydrogen at every available spot in the molecule. In other words, all carbon molecules are "saturated" with hydrogen. If hydrogen molecules are missing, double bonds will be present, and the fat is classified "unsaturated." If one (mono) double bond is present, the fat is a monounsaturated fatty acid. If more than one (poly) double bond is present, it is a polyunsaturated fatty acid. Corn oil, sunflower oil, and safflower oil are all examples of polyunsaturated fats; olive and peanut oil are monounsaturated; butter and lard are saturated. Saturated fats are typically solid (not liquid) at room temperature and found mostly in foods of animal origin. Palm and coconut oil, although found in plants, are highly saturated. They are used extensively by the food industry in such products as commercial cakes and cookies, crackers, cake mixes, nondairy creamers and nondairy whipped toppings. In contrast, unsaturated fats are liquid at room temperature and found solely in foods of plant origin. Fats that are labeled "hydrogenated" or "partially hydrogenated" are examples of plant fats that have been processed in such a way that hydrogen has been added back to the fat to make it solid at room temperature—a desirable characteristic for certain baking purposes.

Cholesterol plays an important role as a structural component of cell membranes and blood lipoproteins (a fat attached to a protein), which transport the lipids in the blood. Bile salts, steroid hormones, and vitamin D—all important in maintaining healthy tissues in the body—are derived from cholesterol (2). Cholesterol is produced by the liver as well as obtained from dietary sources like eggs, cheese, whole milk, and red meats. In healthy persons, the amount of cholesterol synthesized by the liver will decrease to maintain a fairly constant level of cholesterol in the tissues when dietary sources increase.

As mentioned, cholesterol is carried in the blood as part of lipoproteins. Lipoproteins include low density lipoproteins (LDL), and high density lipoproteins (HDL). HDL cholesterol, sometimes referred to as "good" cholesterol, is responsible for transporting cholesterol to the liver, thus preventing the deposit of cholesterol in the arteries. LDL cholesterol, sometimes referred to as "bad" cholesterol, delivers cholesterol to the tissues of the body. As the blood level of LDL cholesterol rises, the cell receptors that help remove the cholesterol from the blood become saturated, causing a rise in blood cholesterol, which enhances the deposition of cholesterol on artery walls.

High HDL ("good") cholesterol concentrations have been shown to have a preventive effect on the development of atherosclerosis. High LDL ("bad") cholesterol concentrations, on the other hand, have been shown to be directly related to an increased incidence of atherosclerosis (1)—the deposition of cholesterol on artery walls which may lead to blockage and result in a heart attack or stroke.

The connection of fats and cholesterol to heart disease is a complex issue, which has been under intensive investigation for decades and no doubt will continue. Studies of various populations of the world have long suggested that high fat diets are associated with increased heart disease (2). In the United States, where heart disease is the number one killer, 1.5 million persons will suffer heart attacks this year, and half will die. More than 300,000 of those who die will be under sixty-five years old (3). A large body of research exists on the relationship of elevated blood cholesterol to heart disease, especially if other risk factors are present. (These are discussed on page 159).

Although controversy among physicians still exists, and many have resisted accepting the benefits of a low fat diet, major efforts are underway to encourage physicians to screen all patients for elevated blood cholesterol and treat first by reducing total fat in the diet. Reducing total fat, especially saturated fat, will reduce blood cholesterol in 50 percent of individuals with an elevated cholesterol level. Reducing cholesterol levels will reduce risk of heart disease, especially if other risk factors are reduced as well (4).

The degree of blood cholesterol reduction in response to a low fat diet varies between individuals and is generally more dramatic the lower the fat intake. The controversy is due in part to the fact that genetic variability between individuals produces conflicting data. For example, the Pima Indians maintain low blood cholesterol levels in spite of a high fat diet. About 10–20 percent of individuals with hypercholesterolemia escape myocardial infarction (heart attack) until the eighth or ninth decade despite high blood cholesterol levels from birth (5). Genetic factors may protect some individuals while causing others to be highly sensitive to the development of atherosclerosis.

Many health professionals have been reluctant to recommend a low fat diet for the entire population precisely because of genetic variance. The ideal situation would be to identify those individuals who are highly sensitive. But it's not known how to do this. It is prudent behavior, therefore, to implement even a few low-fat dietary changes until better diagnostic tools are available.

Total cholesterol in the blood is measured to identify people who may have an increased risk of heart disease. A blood lipoprotein analysis measures not only total cholesterol but LDL, HDL, and other blood fats. This type of analysis is obtained after a twelve-hour fast and is used in conjunction with the results of a physical examination and medical history to determine relative risk for the development of heart disease and to determine the appropriate treatment.

In October 1987, the National Cholesterol Education Program Adult Treatment Panel, sponsored by the National Heart, Lung, and Blood Institute,

Nutrition

released a detailed report to physicians on the detection, evaluation, and treatment of elevated blood-cholesterol levels. The panel of experts, comprised mainly of physicians, recommended (for adults) total blood-cholesterol levels below 200 (milligrams per deciliter) and low density lipoprotein (LDL) cholesterol below 130. Individuals with borderline high blood cholesterol, 200–239 and LDL 130–159, with two other risk factors or definite coronary heart disease, require nutrition management to reduce these levels (4). Blood-cholesterol levels greater than 240 and LDL greater than 160 indicate a high risk for a coronary event—especially if other risk factors are positive (see below). Again, dietary treatment is the cornerstone of therapy and requires at least a six-month trial on the initial, moderate fat-reducing diet referred to as the Step 1 Diet. If the initial trial does not reduce cholesterol levels considerably, a more intensive dietary approach referred to as the Step 2 Diet is indicated before considering drug therapy. If drug therapy is initiated, dietary therapy needs to be continued for maximum benefit. Both are lifetime treatments.

It is important to discuss the other risk factors associated with coronary heart disease. The majority of risk factors are within the patient's control, not the physician's: smoking, obesity, lack of exercise, excessive stress, and diet. Other contributory risk factors included in the National Cholesterol Education Program are being male, hypertension, family history of premature coronary heart disease (definite myocardial infarction or sudden death before age fifty-five in a parent or sibling), low HDL cholesterol, diabetes, and a history of stroke or vascular disease. The goal is to reduce the number and severity of risk factors as much as possible. Individualization of treatment is important, since certain segments of the population—women, the very young, and the very old—may not require as drastic an approach as a man who has suffered a heart attack before age fifty. All risk factors should be taken into account.

Other substances in food may play a role in the prevention of atherosclerosis. The Omega-3 fatty acid found in the high fish diets of Eskimos may be responsible for the low incidence of heart disease among this population, but more research is needed. No one knows how much fish oil high in Omega-3 is safe, let alone necessary to reduce cholesterol levels. In fact, some researchers have found that fish oils actually increase LDL ("bad") cholesterol while decreasing HDL ("good") cholesterol. There simply is not enough data yet to make any recommendations regarding the use of fish oil capsules in the treatment of hypercholesterolemia. The best approach is simply to eat more fish. The richest source of Omega-3 fatty acids include Atlantic mackerel, salmon and herring, bluefish, albacore tuna, halibut, trout, and sardines.

The high olive oil intake of the Mediterranean populations led some researchers to speculate on the protective effect of this monounsaturated fat, since heart disease is low among the Greek and Italian populations. Monounsaturated fatty acids, prevalent in olive and rapeseed (canola) oils, were once thought to have a neutral effect on blood lipids. Several recent human clinical studies suggest that monounsaturated fats may reduce LDL without reducing HDL cholesterol in the blood (6). The National Cholesterol Education Panel recommendations included a higher level of monounsaturated fats than previously recommended. The best sources of monounsaturated fats include olive oils, olives, canola (rapeseed) oil, peanut oil, avocados, and most nuts, with the exception of coconut and walnuts.

Fiber may play a role in reducing blood-cholesterol levels. Specifically, the water-soluble types of fiber, including pectin, guar gum, and oat bran have been shown to lower cholesterol sometimes, whereas bran and cellulose, insoluble forms of fiber, do not (7). Most claims that fiber *supplements* lower cholesterol are unproved. Food sources of fiber are the best choice, with fruits, beans, and oat bran being the best sources of the water-soluble fibers. The isolated fiber found in fiber supplements is not the same as the fiber in food.

Finally, there is exercise. The mechanism for the lipid-lowering effect of exercises is unknown. Aerobic exercise will raise HDL and may lower LDL and total cholesterol—possibly contributing to a decreased risk of heart disease. It does require an intensive approach to obtain the effects mentioned. An individual would need to exercise at his or her target heart rate (60–70 percent of maximum heart rate for age) for a minimum of 30 minutes and up to 60 minutes four to six times per week to produce an increase in HDL and a decrease in LDL (8).

Carbohydrates

Carbohydrates are a group of chemical substances comprised of carbon, hydrogen, and oxygen. Their main function is to provide energy, and they are in fact the body's best source of fuel. Carbohydrates are stored predominantly in the muscle and liver in the form of glycogen. They are categorized as simple or complex. Simple carbohydrates are the sugars like sucrose or table sugar and lactose, the sugar in milk. These sugars are considered "simple" because only one chemical bond must be broken during digestion. The complex carbohydrates, or polysaccharides, consist of long chains of glucose, either branched or unbranched, forming the starches, glycogen, and cellulose. They are considered "complex" because they are large molecules with many chemical bonds which must be broken before the glucose components are available for absorption.

Simple carbohydrates are often referred to as "empty calorie" foods—like sugar, candy, and carbonated, sweetened soft drinks—because they contribute no vitamins, minerals, or protein. They simply provide energy and nothing else. Many wild claims have been made regarding the effects of excessive sugar, from hyperactivity in children to criminal behavior in adults. In fact, the only major health problem that sugar contributes to is the development of dental caries (cavities). Choosing the predominantly complex forms of carbohydrate, which are "nutrient dense"—meaning a substantial number and quantity of nutrients are provided in relationship to the amount of calories—over the simple forms is beneficial.

The best food sources of complex carbohydrates include whole grain breads and cereals, rice, pasta, potatoes, vegetables, fruits, juices, legumes, and all types of whole-grain flour. Cellulose, a form of dietary fiber, is classified as a polysaccharide, or complex carbohydrate. It is the main structural component of plant cell walls. The human body cannot digest cellulose, so the energy it contains is not available. Other polysaccharides also classified as fibers include hemicellulose, pectin, guar gum, and mucilages. Lignin is a noncarbohydrate form of fiber. Fiber is found only in plant sources of food—fruits, vegetables, grains, and legumes. Meat and milk contain no fiber.

Since fiber is undigestible, it technically is not considered a nutrient. However, fiber does seem to play a role in maintaining health, although we are a long way from understanding exactly what that role is.

Each component of fiber has unique chemical and physical properties, which exert different effects on the body. The water-soluble fibers—pectin, gums, and mucilages—lower blood lipids, and thus cholesterol. The food sources of water-soluble fibers include fruits, beans, and oat bran. The insoluble fibers, cellulose, hemicellulose, and lignin, increase fecal weight and decrease transit time through the colon, thus preventing constipation. The best food sources of insoluble fibers include bran cereal, whole grains, and vegetables. The water-absorption property of insoluble fiber, bran specifically, is responsible for the increased weight of the stool and its altered consistency. This is the one universally agreed upon effect of natural fiber (9). It is also generally accepted that fiber decreases pressure within the colon in individuals with increased pressure. The evidence in support of the claim that fiber prevents cancer of the colon and improves the symptoms of diverticular disease and irritable bowel syndrome is much less convincing.

It is unclear how much fiber the diet should contain. Fiber intakes reported from various countries have ranged from 13 grams per day in the United States to 94 grams per day in Mexico. However, because of inadequate data on the chemical composition and the physiological effects of fiber, it is difficult to make a rational, scientific recommendation as to the quantity or type of dietary fiber that should be consumed. Approximations for a desirable fiber intake have ranged from 25 to 50 grams per day.

Enough evidence exists to suggest that Americans should increase their fiber intake (9). It is important to increase fiber in the diet gradually since drastic changes may cause gastrointestinal distress. Adequate fluid intake is equally important when you are increasing the amount of fiber you eat, since a high fiber intake without adequate fluids will cause constipation rather than alleviate it. Fruits and vegetables with washed, edible peelings will increase the fiber content of the diet. It warrants repeating that fiber supplements are not the same as food fiber and (10) should only be used under the direction of a physician. Table 6 provides a list of the average fiber content of food types.

TABLE 5: AVERAGE FIBER CONTENT OF FOOD TYPES*

Legumes, ½ cup, cooked	5 grams
Cereal, bran, ¼ cup	4 grams
Cereal, whole grain, 1 oz.	3 grams
Nuts/seeds, 1 oz.	3 grams
Starchy vegetables, ½ cup (potatoes, brown rice, winter squash)	2 grams
Vegetables, ½ cup	2 grams
Fruit, 1 small piece or ½ cup	2 grams
Breads/crackers, whole grain (1 slice/4 crackers)	2 grams
Meat/fish/poultry	0
Milk/dairy products	0

Environmental Nutrition, October 1986.

Vitamins

The public seems to have an insatiable appetite for phenomenal and sensational stories about nutrition with vitamins as the centerpiece. Vitamins are organic substances needed by the body in minute amounts. Illness can occur when there is a deficiency in vitamin intake. But contrary to what authors of some popular nutrition books would lead us to believe, such illnesses are extremely rare in the United States as well as in most developed countries.

Vitamin supplements are the most abused over-the-counter substance on the market (11). Four out of ten Americans over the age of sixteen take at least one supplement a day. One out of every ten people take five or more supplements daily, and one in seven is classed as a heavy user—consuming an average of nearly eight times the Recommended Daily Allowance (RDA). Annual sales for vitamin and mineral supplements are expected to reach $10 billion by the 1990s. The practice of taking nutrient supplements has become so widespread that four major health organizations, the American Dietetic Association, the American Institute of Nutrition, the American Society for Clinical Nutrition, and the National Council Against Health Fraud, have issued a joint statement warning Americans of the unnecessary and potentially dangerous effects of nutrient supplement use. The FDA has also urged physicians to report any side effects noted in their patients who take megadoses of vitamin and mineral supplements in the same way they report side effects of drugs. The truth is that vitamins and minerals (12) taken in large quantities no longer function as nutrients. They have a pharmacologic effect—that is, they are functioning as a drug. Overdosing with vitamin supplements can result in toxicity symptoms, something very rare when vitamins are consumed in the form of food.

Vitamins are classed according to their solubility in water or fat. The water-soluble vitamins include the B-complex (thiamin, riboflavin, niacin, B_6, folacin, B_{12}) and ascorbic acid (vitamin C). The fat-soluble include vitamins A, D, E, and K. Any excess of the water-soluble vitamins is stored in the liver and fat cells, and so can build up toxic levels.

Water soluble vitamins

New evidence is disproving the notion that water-soluble vitamins are safe in large doses because the excess is excreted. A case in point is vitamin B_6. The RDA for a woman is 2 mg per day but many women have been taking daily doses 1,000 times greater in an attempt to alleviate premenstrual symptoms. As a result, an array of nervous system disorders have been seen, ranging from numbness of the hands and feet to burning and tingling sensations in the skin to muscle incoordination and impaired walking. The symptoms appeared eight months to two years after the patients first began taking megadoses of B_6 supplements (13), and usually subsided gradually when the supplements were discontinued.

The B-complex vitamins speed up various metabolic reactions in the body. Thiamin (B_1), riboflavin (B_2), and niacin help release the energy in foods, while pyridoxine (B_6) is primarily involved in the synthesis of amino acids and the hemoglobin molecule. Folacin is essential for the formation of red blood cells. The conversion of folacin from its inactive to the active form requires vitamin C and niacin and, to a lesser extent, B_6 (1). Vitamin B_{12} (cyanocobalamin) deficiency was discovered to be the cause of pernicious anemia, a fatal disease if not treated. B_{12} is found only in foods of animal origin and requires the intrinsic factor (a protein secreted by the stomach) for absorption.

Ascorbic acid (vitamin C) is required in the formation of collagen, the structural protein of bones, teeth, cartilage, skin, tendons, cornea, and blood vessels (1). Vitamin C also enhances the absorption of iron. Scurvy, the disease due to a lack of vitamin C, is nowadays essentially nonexistent in the United States, except possibly among alcoholics and older people who are unable to care for themselves. Many controversial health claims have been made for megadoses of vitamin C, probably the most famous being that they will prevent the common cold. The research on this question is contradictory and inconclusive, but the value of vitamin C in preventing colds, if any, must be quite limited. On the other hand, large doses of vitamin C can cause problems. They have been identified as adversely affecting copper metabolism, and this may, in turn, cause an increase in blood cholesterol levels. An abrupt discontinuance of large doses of vitamin C has resulted in some cases in what is known as rebound scurvy. This has also occurred in infants whose mothers were taking large quantities of vitamin C during their pregnancy. Although the RDA for vitamin C is 60 mg for adults, less for children, many people take as much as 1,500 mg per day, twenty-six times the RDA. Even higher intakes are not uncommon.

Fat-Soluble Vitamins.

Many people, if asked what the best food source of vitamin A, would probably reply carrots. In fact, carrots contain no vitamin A. Vitamin A is found solely in foods of animal origins such as eggs, butter, liver, and fish oils. Carrots—along with many dark green leafy vegetables and deep yellow/orange fruits and vegetables—do contain beta-carotene, the precursor form of vitamin A. It is desirable to obtain the majority of vitamin A from beta-carotene, because the body will convert as much beta-carotene to vitamin A as it needs, automatically preventing excess storage. Vitamin A is important for growth, vision, especially night vision, and in maintaining healthy skin and mucuous membranes lining the body.

Vitamin D is essential for deposition of calcium and phosphorus in bones and teeth. The main source of vitamin D does not come from food but rather sunlight, which triggers a series of chemical reactions when it strikes the skin. The major food sources include egg yolks, fish-liver oils, and fortified milk. Individuals who have limited exposure to the sun, like coal miners, institutionalized older adults, and people living in far northern areas with long winters and short days, are potentially at risk for vitamin D deficiency. Vitamin D deficiency causes rickets in children and osteomalacia in adults (1). Excessive amounts of this nutrient will result in calcium deposits in soft tissues and abnormally high blood levels of calcium.

Vitamin E, professed for its virile factor and wound-healing properties by many a food faddist, has only been proved to be essential for its protection of the cell from toxic concentrations of oxygen. Sunflower, safflower, corn, and soybean oils are among the best sources of vitamin E.

Vitamin K, named from the Danish word *koagulation*, indicates the vital role this vitamin plays in the blood-clotting process. The best food source of vitamin K is dark-green leafy vegetables. This vitamin is also produced by intestinal bacteria. Antibiotics that kill off these bacteria may cause a deficiency of vitamin K when prescribed for long periods. Newborn infants have been reported with vitamin K deficiency until the intestinal flora is established about a week after birth. Vitamin K is often administered to newborns to prevent hemorrhage.

Vitamins and nutrition.

Clearly the complex and interdependent role of vitamins in maintaining health demonstrates the delicate balance that exists between nutrients and their multiple functions. It is always better to obtain nutrients from foods than from supplements. Vitamins are only part of the nutrition picture, and reliance on nutrient supplements to ensure good nutrition is not a wise practice. Not only is there potential for imbalance but there may be substances present in foods which are important for maintaining health that have not been identified yet. Taking a standard multiple-vitamin supplement, which does not exceed 100 percent of the United States RDA is generally considered a harmless practice. There are, of course, cases when nutrient supplementation is necessary because of impaired absorption, increased needs such as during pregnancy or illness, or a nutrient-drug interaction. Such supplementation should be directed by a knowledgeable physician. Until science provides proof, sensational claims about vitamins should be regarded with considerable skepticism. It is certainly more enjoyable to taste the first ripe strawberries of spring than it is to swallow a 100 mg supplement of ascorbic acid.

TABLE 6: GOOD FOOD SOURCES OF WATER-SOLUBLE VITAMINS

VITAMIN	FOOD SOURCE
Ascorbic acid	Oranges, grapefruits, strawberries, broccoli, tomatoes, potatoes, peppers
Thiamin (B_1)	Lean pork, nuts, whole grains, enriched grain products, beef liver
Riboflavin (B_{12})	Milk, yogurt, cottage cheese, enriched breads, and cereals
Niacin	Fortified cereals, legumes, peanuts meat, poultry, fish, liver
Pyridoxine (B_6)	Liver, lean meats, fish, poultry, whole grains, legumes
Folacin (folic acid)	Leafy green vegetables, yeast, liver
Cyanocobalamin (B_{12})	Meat, fish, poultry, milk

Foods which contain the water-soluble vitamins are especially sensitive to heat, light, and/or exposure to air. To maintain their nutritional value, fruits and vegetables should be consumed as soon as possible after purchase and stored meanwhile in airtight containers. Vegetables should be steamed or boiled in a minimal amount of water just until tender, for maximum nutrient retention. Milk purchased in plastic containers and exposed to light will have a diminished riboflavin content.

Minerals.

Minerals are inorganic substances essential for life; very small quantities are needed. Except for calcium and iron, which have been studied quite extensively, little is known about other minerals like selenium and chromium.

Calcium. One of the most popular minerals of the eighties has been calcium—due, in part, to the marketing efforts of the drug companies. Calcium supplementation has become widespread as women attempt to ward off osteoporosis. The food companies are not wasting any time either. A variety of foods are showing up on grocery-store shelves that have been fortified with calcium. Most of these foods, like orange juice, are typically a very poor source of calcium. Advertisements would lead many of us to believe that we are doomed to develop a hump back and osteoporosis unless we take two 500 mg supplements of calcium daily. This is, to say the least, an oversimplification.

Over 99 percent of calcium in the body is found in the bones and teeth. The other 1 percent is critically important in muscle contraction, blood clotting, nerve signals, activating enzymes, and maintaining the integrity of cell membranes. The body has a number of controlling mechanisms, which maintain calcium levels in the blood. However, there are certain dietary factors which can adversely affect calcium balance in the body. High protein intakes, not unusual for Americans, can increase calcium excretion in the urine (1). Phosphorus, in excess—which may occur when a large quantity of soft drinks, meat, or some antacids are consumed—may decrease body calcium. Absorption of calcium can be increased by a number of dietary factors, including the presence of vitamin D, lactose (milk sugar), and the amino acids lysine and arginine.

Calcium is a prime example of why food is a better source of nutrients than are supplements. The calcium in milk has a number of factors that will enhance its absorption. Milk and its products are an excellent source of calcium, providing 300 mg per 8 ounces of milk or yogurt, 200 mg per 1 ounce of cheese. Adults need about 800 mg daily for maintenance, and children need about 1,200 mg daily to meet the demands of growth. A pregnant woman needs 1,200 mg per day to meet her own needs as well as the needs of the developing fetus. Diets deficient in calcium during pregnancy have resulted in diminished bone density in the newborn. During lactation, 1,200 mg of calcium is still needed daily to prevent maternal demineralization of the bone (14).

Calcium is deposited rapidly in the bones from birth and gradually tapers off around age thirty. If a woman does not consume enough calcium during this phase of her life, her bones will be less dense. A poor calcium intake during the third decade, combined with several pregnancies and breast-feeding, will increase the risk of osteoporosis later in life. Men, who do not experience these losses, are less likely to develop calcium deficiency. Furthermore, large, dense bones are much less likely to become osteoporotic than are small bones. So a man with a large frame has a much smaller risk of having problems than does a petite woman. An increase in calcium intake after age thirty, whether from foods or supplements, will not undo years of suboptimal calcium intake.

The osteroporosis problem is not unique to women, but does have a much higher incidence among postmenopausal women. Bone loss is accelerated when the hormone estrogen diminishes. Estrogen replacement is often prescribed as a means of controlling bone demineralization after menopause.

Zinc deficiency was first identified in 1963. It was found in areas of the Middle East where the diet consists of grains with little or no animal protein. Phytate, a substance in the high grain diet, prevents the absorption of zinc. Marginal zinc deficiency has been found in segments of the United States population as well. Symptoms of zinc deficiency include a failure to grow normally, delayed sexual development, poor appetite, decrease in taste sensitivity, and poor healing of wounds (15). Wound healing and appetite improved in individuals whose low zinc stores were increased. The best sources of zinc are red meat, liver, eggs, and seafood, especially oysters. The RDA for zinc is 15 mg for children over ten years old and adults, 10 mg for children under ten, 20 mg for pregnant women, and 25 mg for women who are breast-feeding (14).

Too much zinc may be detrimental. One study of six healthy men who took twenty times the RDA of zinc for six weeks, found impairment of the white blood cells' ability to fight infection, and increased levels of LDL cholesterol, promoting the risk of cardiovascular disease (15). Excess zinc also interferes with iron function and will aggravate a marginal copper deficiency (15). It is virtually impossible to get too much zinc from food alone, but supplements that exceed the RDA are readily available and are not recommended because serious toxicity and nutrient imbalances may occur.

Iron. The main role of iron in the body is as a component of hemoglobin, which carries oxygen in the blood. Iron occurs in foods in two forms, heme iron found in meats and nonheme iron found in plant sources of food.

Iron deficiency is the most common cause of anemia in the United States.

During periods of rapid growth, as in childhood and adolescence, iron needs are increased. If intake is inadequate, anemia may develop. Women of childbearing age are a high risk group of iron-deficiency anemia, because of monthly blood losses. Pregnancy creates especially high requirements for iron, which cannot be met by diet alone. The RDA is 10 mg for men and postmenopausal women, 18 mg for girls over age ten and women, 30–60 mg for pregnant women. Continuation of 30–60 mg of iron per day for at least two months after childbirth is recommended to replenish maternal iron stores (14).

Sodium is a mineral comprising about 60 percent of table salt. One teaspoon of salt provides 2,300 mg of sodium. There is no RDA for sodium, but in 1980, an Estimated Safe and Adequate Daily Intake was established for sodium by the National Research Council when the RDAs were last revised. Eleven hundred to 3,300 mg per day is recommended for adults, less for children.

In many instances blood pressure is affected by sodium intake. Increasing sodium in the diet tends to increase blood pressure, and reducing sodium tends to lower it. That is why many physicians advise restriction of dietary sodium as one element in a blood-pressure-control program.

Sodium occurs naturally in some foods such as dairy products and seafood, but much is added to foods in processing. Generally, convenience foods like frozen entrees, commercial spaghetti sauce, canned soups, stews, vegetables, cured meats like ham, bacon, hot dogs, bologna, pepperoni, and foods prepared in a brine like pickles, olives, and sauerkraut, are especially high in sodium. Cheese, sausage, bouillon, soy sauce, Worcestershire sauce, and potato chips also rate high on the list. Fruits, fresh or frozen vegetables, whole grain breads and cereals, pasta, rice, bagels, fresh beef, pork, poultry, veal, fish and seafood are typically low or moderate in sodium. For many, the simple elimination of the salt shaker, in both cooking and at the table, will reduce sodium to a more reasonable intake. The use of herbs, spices, flavored vinegars, onions, garlic, lemon, and wine in cooking enhances the taste of foods without killing the natural flavors with salt. There is no known health benefit from excessive sodium intake, and there is a reasonable possibility that a low salt intake, established early in life and continued, may prevent (in the 20 percent of children who are at risk) hypertension later in life (14). Sodium content has been required on food labels since July 1986 and is listed in mg per serving.

Potassium, like sodium, helps the body maintain fluid balance. It also plays a key role in maintaining the pH balance, nerve transmission, and muscle contraction, especially that of the heart muscle. Bananas and orange juice are most frequently named as the best sources of potassium. In fact, potassium is widespread throughout the food supply from dairy products to meats, fish, poultry, fruits, and vegetables.

Potassium deficiency is usually associated with excessive losses from diarrhea, vomiting, laxative abuse, and as a side effect of some diuretics. Toxicity can result in cardiac arrest. For this reason, potassium supplements should be used only under the direction of a physician.

Some individuals with hypertension who are avoiding salt and salty foods prefer to use a salt substitute. Salt substitutes are either a combination of sodium and potassium or entirely potassium chloride. Excessive intake of potassium from salt substitutes usually does not occur, as too much causes a bitter taste. However, for someone taking potassium supplements, use of a salt substitute may increase the risk of potassium toxicity. Some medications cause the body to retain potassium. Use of salt substitutes with such medication is another possible cause of potassium toxicity. The Estimated Safe and Adequate Daily Dietary Intake for potassium is 1,875 to 5,625 mg for adults (14).

Water. Water is the most critical of all nutrients. Death from water deprivation occurs in days, whereas it may take months before death occurs from starvation. The body consists of 50–75 percent water, depending on age and percentage of body fat. About 2 liters (slightly more than 2 quarts) of water is lost each day through urine, feces, perspiration, and expired air. This fluid (64 ounces) needs to be replaced everyday; hence the rationale for eight 8-ounce glasses of water per day. Fluid intake and output accounts for the daily fluctuations in body weight. Water is important in maintaining body temperature, transporting nutrients to and from the cells, multiple chemical reactions, and cellular metabolism. The main sources of water, other than drinking water, include all beverages, fruits, and vegetables.

OBESITY: THEORIES AND MYTHS

Obesity, defined as being 20 percent or more above one's desirable weight, afflicts over 34 million Americans. Morbid obesity is 100 pounds overweight or 100 percent over ideal weight. Obesity, in general, is associated with heart disease, hypertension, hypercholesterolemia, cancer, pulmonary, endocrine, and digestive disorders, rheumatoid arthritis, and psychological disorders.

Originally, it was thought that fat people simply ate too much. Indeed for many it is a matter of an energy imbalance caused by a consistent intake of calories exceeding energy requirements. In other words, the energy input (food) exceeds the energy output (exercise plus basal metabolic needs plus the energy to digest food). However, research and knowledge have progressed beyond the simple generalizations of the past. Obesity is now thought to be a complex disease, having multiple causes and of different types (16-18).

A number of theories on the causes of obesity have been proposed over the years. Of particular interest is the fat cell theory. Research has indicated that the body increases the number of fat cells at different times during the life cycle, with the prime time occurring from birth to age five and again from seven to eleven (19). Overfeeding in infancy and childhood may indeed predispose an individual to the development of obesity later in life, because of additional fat cells. Once a fat cell develops, it is there for life. The size of the cells may decrease in response to weight reduction, but the same number of fat cells still exist. Obese people tend to have fat cells that are two to two and a half times larger than normal-weight persons.

Metabolism also plays into the fat-cell theory. Consider the chronic dieter, who repeatedly takes drastic measures to lose weight quickly, such as very-low-calorie diets, very-low-carbohydrate diets, liquid diets, or semistarvation diets. The first fast drop in weight results from the loss not only of fat, but of water and lean muscle tissue. The water loss is temporary. Lean muscle tissue is metabolically more active than fat, meaning it takes more energy (calories) to maintain a muscle cell than a fat cell. If you lose muscle, your base-line caloric needs decrease, making it that much harder to lose weight. (19).

Consider an obese woman who decides to reduce her calorie intake drastically. The body interprets this as a state of starvation and will conserve all energy by slowing down its metabolic needs (20). It's a protective mechanism to prevent death, probably leftover from early times when man was a hunter and gatherer and would have to go for long periods of time without food. After a few weeks, the dieter can no longer tolerate this monotonous, impractical dietary regimen and reverts back to previous eating habits. Originally she only needed about 1,500 calories a day to maintain her state of overweightedness. At less than 1,000 calories daily, she did lose weight but at the expense of decreasing her metabolic needs. Now she only needs 1,200 calories to maintain her weight, but she is eating 2,500 calories per day and rapidly regaining the few pounds she lost plus more. As a result, what she lost as lean muscle tissue is now being replaced by more fat cells. Each time she attempts weight loss in this manner, she may become fatter than she was to begin with, perpetuating the process. Considering the negative consequences of improper weight loss regimens, it may be more appropriate for an overweight person to work at maintaining his current weight than to fall victim to the cycle described and possibly become even heavier and fatter.

When the fat cells of a group of normal-weight people who had previously all been over 200 pounds were examined, it was found that their body chemistries were abnormal. Their fat cells resembled the fat cells of a starving person. They were extremely tiny. The women no longer menstruated, their pulse rates and blood pressures were low. They were always cold, and they burned 25 percent fewer calories than would be expected on the basis of their heights and weights. The cells not only looked biochemically like the cells of starving people, but the individuals studied acted like it, always thinking about food, and many working in the weight-loss business (17). For some obese people, a "normal" weight may be biologically abnormal. This biologically abnormal state may pressure the body to refill the empty fat cells. The fat-cell theory may explain why so many people who have successfully lost weight are unable to keep from regaining it.

Another aspect of the fat-cell theory has to do with small molecules on the surfaces of fat cells known as alpha and beta receptors. The alpha receptors stimulate fat accumulation, and the beta receptors stimulate the breakdown of fat. Human fat cells have both of these receptors but one is more dominant. Women tend to have fat cells with predominantly alpha receptors, fat accumulators, on their hips and thighs. Men carry most of their alphs receptors in the abdomen. This explains why some people who embark on a weight-loss program lose weight, but not where they intend to lose it most.

Yet another popular explanation is known as the set-point theory. This theory maintains that the body has a unique, relatively stable adult weight, determined by various biological factors. Two important human studies demonstrated that the body will return to its biologically natural weight in spite of dietary manipulation causing weight loss or gain (19, 20). In other words, the body controls its weight somewhat the same way that a thermostat controls temperature. Some proponents of this theory have suggested methods to alter the body's set point to a lower weight. Much more research on the set-point theory is required before a safe method is determined effective.

A number of other factors play a role in contributing to one's weight status throughout the life cycle, including age, sex, body size, genetics, and exercise. As we age, our metabolism slows down—about 2 percent per decade beginning with the third decade (14). Energy needs are at their highest from infancy through young adulthood, because these are the growing years. Men generally have a higher BMR (basal metabolic rate) than women do, partly because of size and body composition. Women have a higher percentage of body fat, approximately 20–22 percent compared to men who have 12–15 percent body fat (if they are of normal weight). Energy requirements are directly related to size. The bigger a person is, the more energy he needs to maintain his size. Both body composition and size contribute to the fact that obesity is more common in women than men (19).

The tendency for obesity to run in families has long been noted. Recent research results have suggested that a genetic predisposition to obesity is highly probable (20), but environment obviously contributes to this process also. A child with the genetic predisposition to obesity, living in a permissive eating environment, is more likely to become an obese adult than if the same child were living in a controlled eating environment. However, even in families where obesity is common, it is not necessarily inevitable.

Possibly of greatest importance in weight control are the effects of activity (21). Activity does not necessarily have to be in the form of an exercise regimen, although an appropriate exercise program is likely to be more efficient in weight reduction and control when combined with a safe nutrition program. For people who are unable and/or unwilling to initiate an exercise program, or maintain one, adding activities to their habits of daily living can contribute to a very slow but significant weight loss without substantial calorie reduction. Consider taking the stairs instead of the elevator, parking farther from the office building, grocery store, or movie theater, and thus walking more and burning more calories. Reevaluate what trips can be done on foot instead of in the car. The importance of regular activity cannot be overemphasized. The benefits are numerous. In addition to promoting loss of weight while increasing lean muscle tissue, exercise has positive effects on the heart, lungs, blood pressure, pulse, and metabolism.

Selecting a safe nutrition program and combining it with a safe exercise program is the best approach for effective, permanent weight loss. Behavior management is essential for long-term success. Group support may or may not be beneficial, depending on the individual. Consultation with a registered dietitian (R.D.) is strongly recommended. The following characteristics are representative of a safe weight-loss program.

- The foundation of the diet is based on a wide variety of foods, including all of the basic four food groups, readily available in any grocery store. Food choices are made by the individual, not from preplanned menus.

- Weight is measured no more than twice a week. Daily weights will reflect fluid changes, not fat loss, and are a self-defeating behavior. The lowest weight will be in the morning, before eating or drinking, after the bladder is emptied, nude.

- A goal or ideal weight is determined by measuring height, wrist circumference for bone structure, preferably skin folds for percentage of body fat, and actual weight without shoes. The individual's weight history and age need to be taken into account as well. Some people have never weighed their "desirable weight" (according to the life insurance weight tables), and it is unrealistic to set such weight goals. Weight tables are only minimally useful, because women, the poor, and minorities were underrepresented in their compiling (the majority of people who purchase life insurance are white upper-class males). The validity of the Metropolitan Weight Tables, for example, is further questioned because the effects of smoking and age were not taken into account. In some cases, heights and weights were self-reported, not actually measured.

- Weight loss should not exceed 1–2 pounds per week. A faster weight loss will result in a greater loss of lean muscle tissue and water, which is undesirable and potentially dangerous. A rate of weight loss greater than 2 pounds per week should be monitored on a regular basis by a knowledgeable physician.
- Calorie requirements are highly individualized, but in general should not be less than 1,200 calories per day for women and not less than 1,500 calories per day for men. A registered dietitian individualizes diet prescriptions on the basis of size, age, and activity level. Individuals who choose weight-loss programs of less than 1,200 calories per day should be under the direction of a knowledgeable physician, because there is a potential risk of metabolic imbalances and nutritional deficiencies.
- Vitamin and mineral supplements as well as protein powders, bee pollen, lecithin, or any other nutritional supplement are not necessary and are not recommended. If the nutrition component is safe and balanced, supplements are a waste of money and potentially harmful at doses exceeding the Recommended Daily Dietary Allowances. Unless there is an established deficiency, nutrients should be obtained from foods. If a weight-loss program requires use of supplements, it should be interpreted as a warning that the diet itself is inadequate, imbalanced, and/or unlikely to work for a lifetime.
- Inclusion of a safe exercise program is essential.
- Methods for identifying improper eating behaviors and specific means of altering those habits permanently is also an essential component. Motivational techniques, positive thinking, support systems, and relapse prevention strategies provide important tools to enhance success.
- Emphasis is on reducing fat to no more than 30 percent of the calories: protein should comprise between 15 and 20 percent of the calories from lean sources; and carbohydrates, predominantly complex, high-fiber types, should comprise the remaining 50–55 percent of calories.
- Planning for holidays, special occasions, parties, and eating out is important, for the individual should be able to participate without feeling guilty and without regaining weight. At holiday time there will always be more food available than usual. The trick is to plan for the event and be prepared to exercise more frequently before, during, and/or after the event.
- Information on portion control, low-fat cooking methods, grocery shopping, and food-label interpretation is available, to provide the individual with a greater ability to make consistently wise food choices.
- An option to include small quantities of sweets, alcohol, and/or favorite high-fat/high-calorie foods is important for some individuals. Such an occasional indulgence helps prevent feelings of deprivation, which often lead

to overindulgence. No food or foods should be "forbidden." It's important to think in terms of frequency and quantity. The dieter should feel that he or she can live with his nutrition program for life. If the person is satisfied and does not think of himself as "on a diet," long-term weight control becomes integrated into the individual's life-style and requires a less conscious effort, becoming more automatic.

- The Golden Rule: "If it's not in the house, you can't eat it." As simple as this rule sounds, it is amazingly effective. For example, people who have a problem with sweets will be in trouble if there are ice cream in the freezer, cookies in the cabinet, chocolates in candy dishes around the house. If these types of foods are no longer brought home from the store, the dieters will avoid temptation. It's better to plan to have sweets when you go out to eat, because the quantity is controlled, and once the cake or pie is eaten, it's gone. Half of it isn't sitting on the counter, beckoning to you.

- Psychological readiness and attitude are two important factors an individual needs to consider seriously before embarking on a weight-loss program. If he is not really ready, he may fight himself for weeks or months, feeling completely miserable, and still not lose much weight. Periods of high stress are not conducive to making life-style changes, and for you the time may be a critical element. A weight-loss program started in December will probably not go very far. During times of stress or during holidays and vacations, it might be better to choose a more realistic goal, like controlling weight instead of losing weight.

In spite of all the serious health problems associated with obesity, health is not the motivating factor for the majority of people who want to lose weight. Psychosocial problems may rank as far more compelling. This appears to be especially true for women. The psychological burden of obesity is enormous, as is seen in the statistics of anorexia nervosa and bulimia. It is estimated that 95 percent of bulimics are female (22). Anorexia and bulimia combined affect 5 to 15 percent of all adolescent girls and teenagers (22).

We are a nation obsessed with thinness and dieting. The emaciated look of the New York high-fashion model is set as an ideal body image. The cure is as complex as the cause. For many obese people, including children and teenagers, the cause is intertwined with family problems, stressful life events, behavioral, psychological, medical, and genetic factors. Despite the common belief by health professionals that fewer than 5 percent of obese individuals achieve and maintain their goal weight, the reality is much more optimistic (23). Many people who have successfully lost and maintained weight on their own have not been included in the statistics. Nor do the statistics represent new developments in treatment that produce greater and longer-lasting weight losses. As the prevalence of obesity grows, so will the knowledge and the optimism to treat it successfully.

WHAT IS A NUTRITIONIST?

A great deal of confusion exists regarding what a nutritionist actually is and isn't. Essentially there are two major types of nutritionists; the qualified nutritionist and the self-proclaimed nutritionist. Although not all qualified nutritionists are "registered dietitians," the majority are. An R.D. has met specific education, training, and testing requirements established by the Commission on Dietetic Registration of the American Dietetic Association. They include a minimum of a B.S. in food and nutrition from an accredited university, completion of an ADA-approved dietetic internship (usually nine to twelve months), and passing a nationally administered registration exam. This is the most common route to becoming registered, but there are other options. Whichever route she chooses, after passing her exam, the R.D. must pay dues annually to the ADA and maintain seventy-five continuing-education credits per five-year period. There are over 40,000 registered dietitians in the United States.

Some qualified nutritionists choose not to be registered: food scientists, Ph.D. nutritionists, B.S.-and M.S.-level nutritionists. Some home economists consider themselves nutritionists, since portions of their curricula do overlap. More recently physicians have been specializing in nutrition, usually in addition to board certification as a family practitioner or gastroenterologist.

The qualified nutritionist has completed in-depth education and training in nutrition, over a period of four to six and a half years. In contrast, the self-proclaimed nutritionist usually has had no formal training in the science of nutrition at all. Many may simply have developed an interest in the subject after reading a few popular books. Or, as is also common, an individual has a weight problem and after losing 20 pounds at a weight-loss franchise, decides to become a counselor. Many people who work in this capacity incorrectly call themselves nutritionists. They sell "nutrition" on the basis of what the franchise tells them to say. Scientifically unproved claims may be mixed with facts.

Many weight loss panaceas have been promoted by the pyramid sales scheme. Each buyer of the new product is encouraged to become a seller and proselytizer also. In this way sales "pyramid" with minimal overhead and minimal accountability. The product might be, for example, a powdered form of nutriment, highly fortified with "everything you need." Such products are often marketed for weight loss, weight gain, weight maintenance, achieving optimal health, etc. Sound too good to be true? The company may develop a very slick marketing approach, promising an effortless approach to weight loss—especially appealing to the obese person who has struggled with excess weight for years. Anyone may be recruited to sell these products, no education or training in nutrition required—you only have to learn how to sell the product. At best, this situation usually results in financial loss as these products are expensive. At worst, the customers may suffer physically, either from adverse effects of the product itself or from delay in obtaining medical treatment, because they were led to believe the product would cure all their pains and ailments. The companies often cover themselves by saying they never told their sales people to make unsubstantiated health claims about their product, which may very well be true. When the FDA attempts to follow up on a complaint about a specific product, they often are unable to find out who actually sold the product and what false claims were made, since the customers who were harmed may be reluctant to identify their neighbor, friend, or relative as the culprit. These companies have a strong profit motive, not a health-care motive.

Also of concern are *some* health food stores. These are much used sources of vitamin supplements and various so-called health foods such as herbal teas and exotic African plants. Various unsubstantiated claims of benefit such as relief of pain, improvement in skin textures, and so on are often made. Most of the products are probably harmless, but also useless and very expensive. These stores may be managed by and patronized by self-proclaimed nutritionists.

The situation is further complicated by the endless stream of popular nutrition books, all promising effortless weight loss, disease prevention, longevity, and your basic cure-all, through yet another interpretation of nutrition. Qualified nutritionists spend as much time undoing myths and wild notions about food and nutrition as they do educating people on the facts. Indeed much of the nutrition information published is written by the do-it-yourself nutritionist. Although "Dr." is often tagged onto the names of these people, the first question should be "doctor of what?" Is the degree from an accredited university or from a mail-order diploma mill? If the degree is genuine, is it even remotely related to nutrition? (In fact, a recently published nutrition book advised the reader how to be his own nutritionist.)

How does one tell then the difference between a qualified nutritionist and a potential fraud? Well, first look for the initials R.D. or L.D. "licensed dietician") after the name. The title "registered dietitian" is protected by the American Dietetic Association and cannot legally be used by anyone who has not met, and continues to meet, the requirements established by the ADA. Ask about education, training, and experience. Unfortunately for both the public and qualified nutritionists, only a few states have established mandatory licensure regulating dietitians/nutritionists. Considering that such professionals as beauticians and morticians, electricians and realtors, are regulated by licensing laws, it is amazing that the licensure of nutritionists has met with such resistance.

A number of characteristics common to self-proclaimed nutritionists may help you to distinguish between them and true professionals. Assertions that sound too good to be true are often exactly that: unsubstantiated claims for great benefits from eating "organic foods," megadoses of vitamins, and fad diets. Or too bad to be true: unsubstantiated claims about the dangers of various additives and preservatives. Problems with our food supply do exist, but in general the American diet is still probably the richest, most varied, and safest in the world—in part because of those much-maligned additives, which among other things protect the consumer by preventing the spoilage of food. All additives ought to be evaluated on the basis of scientific evidence, not name calling.

Who Needs a Nutritionist?

The people who need a nutritionist can be divided into two categories: those who are healthy and those who have medical problems that require nutrition intervention. The latter group includes people who have diabetes, heart disease, high blood pressure, cancer, kidney failure, gastrointestinal problems, food allergies, and eating disorders. Individuals who have medical problems complicated by obesity would also benefit. Nutrition services and care are considered an adjunct to medical treatment, not a substitute. However, in certain medical problems like noninsulin dependent diabetes and hypercholesterolemia (high blood cholesterol), nutrition management may be the cornerstone of treatment.

But even most healthy people have room for improvement when it comes to their food choices and eating habits, whether they need to decrease fat, increase fiber, lose weight, or gain weight. Getting the facts from a qualified nutritionist and applying the recommendations to one's life-style may have a significant impact on lifelong health. A good example is the person who has a positive family history for hypercholesterolemia and heart disease. If he or she establishes a low-fat eating style, it might minimize major health problems down the road.

The following list highlights those segments of the healthy population who may be in need of a nutritionist:

1. Women planning to become pregnant (preconceptual nutrition).
2. Pregnant women (prenatal nutrition, recommended during the first trimester).
3. Vegetarians or people considering a vegetarian eating style.
4. Athletes, professional or nonprofessional.

5. Individuals and families with a positive family history for heart disease, hypertension, or cancer.
6. People with weight problems, moderate to severe—childhood, adolescent, or adult.
7. Business people who travel and eat in restaurants frequently and anyone who eats out on a daily basis.

Like doctors, dietitians have been specializing in various areas, such as critical care, pediatrics, maternal and infant nutrition, heart disease, sports nutrition, and wellness. Many dietitians work as generalists and have a wide range of experience to draw from.

What to Expect?

A responsible, qualified nutritionist will obtain information on your eating habits, portion sizes, food preparation, life-style, medical history, weight history, previous diet prescriptions by physicians, previous weight-loss attempts, prescription and nonprescription medicines, use of nutrient supplements, family history for disease, bowel habits, food allergies or intolerances, activity level and exercise habits, results of pertinent blood work or other medical tests, if available.

On the basis of the above information, the nutritionist will design an individualized nutrition program to fit your unique nutrition needs. The program should include recommendations for the occasional treat: favorite foods, alcohol, dining out, snacking, and planning for holidays and parties. Preprinted diets without individualized counseling are not the sign of a qualified nutritionist. In short, the program should be one the individual can live with for life. Emphasis on obtaining nutrients from food, including a wide variety of foods, behavior-modification techniques, and exercise should also be included. Adequate time for education and questions should be provided as well as appropriate materials. The professional nutritionist will encourage a positive and supportive climate to facilitate an open rapport, learning, and dietary change.

NUTRITION IN PERSPECTIVE

Food and nutrition mean different things to different people. It is associated with our earliest feelings of bonding with our parents. It is part of many memories of happy family and social events. It is part of our ethnic heritage. In its purest form, food is sustenance.

Food alone cannot cure or prevent illness, but food is one of several factors that contribute to developing and maintaining health. It becomes a matter of choice: How *consistently* wise are our food choices?

We need not make perfect food choices 100 percent of the time. This is not realistic. The dieter who swears never to eat a piece of cake or cookies again sets himself up for failure. Looking at the total picture, not just one part, helps to put food and nutrition in perspective. If the quality of food choices are 85–90 percent on target 85–90 percent of the time, that is excellent. If not, that is a nutrition goal to work toward.

Human beings are creatures of habit, not the least of which is eating. Because eating habits are ingrained early in life, they are among the toughest to change. And it's not a habit we can eschew entirely, like smoking—we must eat everyday. Therefore we must make changes within certain prescribed limits and stick to those changes. Patience is as important as perspective in reforming bad eating habits. Expecting too much too soon does not allow the brain time to adapt to changes we are making. A positive attitude, patience, and perspective will go a long way toward enhancing health through optimal nutrition.

8

STAYING HEALTHY
Kurt Link, M.D.

One narrow definition of health is the absence of disease. In many ways this is an inadequate view of health, but to keep things simple, let us use this definition here. Health maintenance, like every other area of medical practice, is characterized by uncertainty and controversy, speculation, theorizing, hypothesis, inconsistencies and contradictions. But in this chapter I am going to emphasize those aspects of health maintenance that have been either scientifically proved or at least widely accepted by experts. I will put aside the great temptation to speculate about issues, and I will try to present what is known, which accounts for the brevity of this chapter.

What follows applies to healthy adults not known to be at unusual risk for any particular illness. These standard rules and recommendations may not apply if you have a chronic illness such as diabetes, high blood pressure, or emphysema, if you are pregnant, if you have a family history of a hereditary disease, if you have any unusual occupational exposures or hazards. In all those cases, there may be specific preventive measures that you should take that are not appropriate for the general population.

LIFE-STYLE

Whether or not you stay healthy is largely in your own hands. There are some factors, such as your heredity, over which you have no control. But you can control other factors that have a great impact on your health. Your life-style is the key to staying healthy and is far more important than medical care. Let us review some of the more practical aspects of a healthy life-style.

Cigarettes. There is not much to say about cigarettes. Everybody knows that they cause lung cancer and heart attacks. They also cause chronic bronchitis and emphysema, cancer of the mouth, bladder, and kidney; hardening of the arteries that sometimes leads to gangrene and amputations, strokes, complications of pregnancy, peptic ulcer. In America, cigarette smoking is the most important single cause of preventable death (1). Those who want to do so can paint this black and white picture gray, and say, "Yes, but . . ." or "There are other factors involved." Everybody knows somebody who smoked every day of his life and lived to be ninety-four. But the man or woman dying of lung cancer is almost always a cigarette smoker. The man laid low by a heart attack at age forty-two is almost always a cigarette smoker, and so is the person with half his face gone to mouth cancer. All the checkups and chest X-rays in the world can't protect you from the risk you take by smoking cigarettes.

Many experts on cigarette smoking consider it an addiction. There is little doubt that physical addiction to nicotine does occur. The nicotine chewing gum (Nicorette) can help with that part of the habit, and support and self-help groups and a variety of smoke-cessation programs can help you desire to be a nonsmoker. Many smokers, even hard-core two- or three-pack-a-day smokers, do quit. The smarter ones do it *before* their heart attacks.

Alcohol. Alcoholism is discussed in the chapter on addiction. Small amounts of alcohol, such as an ounce of liquor or 8 ounces of beer or wine, are generally considered not to be harmful. But it is impossible to define a safe level, because there is great individual variation in susceptibility to the harmful effects of alcohol. Some heavy drinkers never have ill effects; other moderate social drinkers develop heart failure or cirrhosis of the liver. And even small amounts of alcohol can be dangerous if you are driving, swimming, operating machinery, etc. If you have any adverse effects from alcohol, be they related to injuries, your health, your work, personal relationships, or problems with the law, then you are drinking too much. If there is any doubt, the safe and prudent thing to do is to stop.

Illegal drugs. The hard drugs are also discussed in the chapter on addiction. Today using any injectable street drug is frankly suicidal behavior. Cocaine in all its forms can also cause serious and sometimes fatal complications. Marijuana smoking can cause the same harmful effects as cigarettes and psychological and socially adverse effects as well.

Sexually transmitted disease. Your risk of contracting a sexually transmitted disease depends entirely on your sexual activities. AIDS can be transmitted in many ways, one of which is through sex. In this country the most common form of sexual transmission is via unprotected passive anal intercourse among homosexuals, but any intimate contact, homosexual or heterosexual, which transfers bodily fluids, can transmit the responsible virus. Gonorrhea, syphilis, and herpes are less deadly but more common than AIDS. All of these conditions can be prevented by celibacy or strictly monogamous sexual relationships. Moreover, even the sexually active person with more than one partner (or a partner with more than one partner) is unlikely to become infected if there is no rectal sex, if there are few partners, and if condoms are used. Individuals with many sex partners are at increasing risk, especially if the partners are homosexual, bisexual, or IV drug users. If you are in a high risk group or suspect that you have been exposed to a sexually transmitted disease, a visit to your doctor for appropriate examinations, blood test, and cultures is in order.

Injuries. Injury is the leading cause of death for people between the ages of one and forty-five years. Prevention of deaths due to injuries is "the sleeping giant of preventive medicine" (2). The regular use of automobile seatbelts is perhaps the best-documented method of preventing injuries, but every adult can create a safer environment for himself and loved ones. In eliminating injuries from auto accidents, seatbelts are only one factor. You should drive only when you are alert and when mirrors, steering, brakes, and other safety features are in order, and you should try to avoid driving in dangerous weather conditions. In the house, stairs should be free of obstructions and should have handrails, especially important for elderly persons. Falls in bathtubs can also be prevented by handholds and nonslip surfacing. Tools, especially power tools, should be used only with appropriate goggles, boots, gloves, dust masks, and safety devices. Injuries are among the leading causes of death of young people; 1.4 percent of all American boys, aged fifteen to twenty-five, will die of an injury. Half of all deaths from unintended injury are due to automobile and motorcycle traffic. Falls, drowning, and fires are the next most common causes. Many times the injured person was not to blame—merely the innocent victim of an unavoidable incident—but many accidents are avoidable, such as those connected with excessive alcohol use, inadequate supervision of teenagers, failure to use seatbelts, and lack of a safe environment for the elderly.

Exercise. There is considerable evidence that exercise is good for you. Exercise decreases the body's need for insulin and may lower blood fats; it tends to strengthen bones and prevent osteoporosis; many exercisers believe that they have more self-confidence and higher energy levels than they used to have and are better able to tolerate stress. But in fairness to those who prefer repose to exertion, it should be noted that there is no real proof that exercise prevents heart attacks, results in less illness, better mental health, or longer life span.

To achieve such benefits as may be produced by exercise, the Kevin Cooper aerobics formula still holds true: Maximum benefit requires the equivalent of at least 30 minutes of exercise that raises the pulse rate to about 75 percent or your maximum heart rate (220 minus your age), and this must be done at least three times a week. Extremists, like marathon runners (among

Staying Healthy

whom I number), are not exercising for health; they may have neurotic needs or be on a semispiritual quest to seek the limits of their endurance or capabilities. Physical injuries due to trauma or overuse, heat injuries, endocrine disturbances, and other ill effects are common in this group, and some members suffer from psychological disturbances as well.

Diet. Nutrition has been discussed in detail in another chapter. The basic rules for a good diet are simple. If you have no special needs and are on no medication, the rules are these: three meals a day, with selections from the three major food groups; some fresh fruits and vegetables; not too many calories; avoid foods high in sodium and keep away the salt shaker; minimize animal and dairy fats but get plenty of calcium in early adulthood (especially women, more especially mothers): include fiber. To this you need add no additives, no vitamins, no "health" foods.

Overweight. Obesity as a problem in nutrition is discussed in the nutrition chapter. In this chapter let us look at obesity as a medical problem. Most overweight people think they know about the adverse effects of being overweight; they should, because from childhood, parents, peers, teachers, and above all doctors have been telling them how sick they are or will soon be. It turns out, however, that the greatest adverse effect of obesity is its psychological burden (3), to which the constant harangues by others contribute.

I am speaking here of mild to moderate obesity. (Severe obesity, known in the medical literature as "morbid" obesity—defined as greater than 100 pounds overweight or more than double your normal weight—is a serious medical problem.) Even ordinary obesity in and of itself does put you at risk for certain ailments, but these risks are commonly much exaggerated. The connection between overweight and heart attacks, for example, is very uncertain. In fact the evidence does *not* support the hypothesis that obesity causes atherosclerosis (4). Many, indeed most, fat people are not sick—they feel fine, have normal blood pressure, blood sugar, and cholesterol. Nonetheless, most fat people are forever trying to lose weight. The observable fact is, however, that most will not lose weight and succeed in keeping it off. This is not because they are of a poor character. If you are overweight and diet to lose weight, your body reacts as if it were starving (4); you are pitting your will against the call of your body. With some exceptions, mystics and fanatics are the only ones who win such contests.

If you are obese and can't lose weight, take extra care to do everything possible to prevent the possible complications of obesity. Don't smoke. Do exercise. Fat people can be good athletes. Swimming is the overweight athlete's forte, but overweight people can also ride bikes, jog, and participate in other sports. If your blood pressure is up, make sure you get it down—by salt restriction, exercise, meditation, or medication. If your cholesterol is too high, get *it* down the same way. If you are obese and have surgery, you are more likely to develop bloodclots (thrombophlebitis) in the veins in your legs postoperatively. So make sure your surgeon uses one of the methods known to prevent such blood clots. There appears to be a connection between obesity and certain cancers, especially of the female organs, so keep up to date on your gynecologic exams and PAP smears.

IMMUNIZATIONS

Immunization is the crown jewel of modern preventive medicine. Immunization is so easy and effective that it tends to be taken for granted and forgotten, especially by adults and physicians who care for adults. In the chapter on medications, I reviewed in some detail the risks and benefits of some vaccines. Here I will simply note the widely accepted recommendations for immunizations of adults. If you want more information, there is a publication (5) by the American College of Physicians that has a detailed discussion of adult immunization recommendations. For purposes of this discussion, I will assume that the usual childhood vaccines have been given. See the discussion of DPT and the other vaccines (page 87) about some controversies in this area.

Tetanus. Tetanus is a fatal infection caused by bacteria normally found in soil. Booster shots are needed every ten years to maintain a high level of immunity. If you have not had a tetanus shot in over ten years, or if you do not know when you last had one, you should get a booster. Tetanus is usually coadministered with diphtheria toxoid, which also wears off in about ten years. So the usual booster is the Td (adult type) toxoid.

Rubella. All persons should be immune to rubella (German measles), but especially health-care workers and women of childbearing age, because rubella, which is usually not a serious disease in children or adults, can be devastating to a fetus. If you have been vaccinated after the age of one, you can assume that you are immune. (Vaccination before age one may not be effective). If you are unsure about having been vaccinated, blood tests can be done to see if you are immune or not. If you are not immune, or if you don't want to take the blood test, you should get vaccinated. The rubella vaccine is commonly combined with measles and mumps vaccine (MMR), and is usually administered in that combination. Of course a young woman taking the vaccine must be certain that she is not pregnant and will not become pregnant for the next three months.

Measles. Those of us born before 1957 can safely assume that we are immune; virtually *everyone* got measles. If you were born after 1957 and received the live measles vaccine when at least one-year-old, you too can assume that you are immune. Between 1963 and 1967 a killed measles vaccine was sometimes used. If you received such a vaccine, or don't know what kind of vaccine you received during those years, you may not be immune. Also, if you were immunized before twelve months of age, you may not be immune. If there is any question about your immune status, you can have the antibody test done to find out, or you can just go ahead and get the vaccine (usually given with the mumps and rubella vaccine [MMR]).

Influenza. This vaccine has had some bad press because of adverse reactions associated with the swine flu vaccine of 1978–79. Other problems are created by the virus itself. It changes every year, so manufacturers constantly have to produce new vaccines. In some years, the variant causing most of the cases of flu is not the one anticipated, so the vaccine may be ineffective.

Nonetheless, the flu vaccine is usually protective. The vaccine is strongly recommended for those at risk for complications: over age sixty-five and those with chronic illnesses such as lung disease or heart trouble. Health-care workers and nursing-home residents should also get the vaccine. It is optional for the younger and otherwise healthy.

Pneumococcal disease. That ancient germ, the pneumococcus, is the cause of perhaps the most common form of bacterial pneumonia. It can also cause meningitis and other serious infections. Infection with the pneumococcus is most common in persons over forty, and these are the persons most likely to die from it. Individuals with impaired immune defenses, with chronic disease such as diabetes, heart failure, or emphysema, and individuals who have lost their spleen are also vulnerable. All such persons should take the pneumococcus vaccine.

THE PERIODIC CHECKUP

The annual physical, which seems so logical and sensible, has come upon hard times. It turns out that the annual physical is largely a costly ritual that has no demonstrable benefit. That discovery has come as a shock to many doctors and patients, but the accumulated evidence has become incontrovertible. A few (very few) aspects of the preventive health examination are definitely valuable. There are some other tests that are widely accepted as useful even though vigorous proof of their value is lacking. There is controversy and uncertainty about even the best of tests. Experts even disagree, for example, about how often and at what ages the PAP smear and mammogram should be done.

With these thoughts in mind, I make the recommendations that follow. These are based on my own practice and a study of the literature. However, let me repeat the qualification that I made at the beginning of this chapter: These recommendations for preventive care apply only to healthy people who have no symptoms or known illness, and who do *not* belong to any high risk group.

Some of the tests and examinations listed below are costly, and incredibly many private and government health insurances do not pay for preventive medicine. (See Chapter 3.) This is a difficult problem that can only be solved by political pressure from informed and aggressive citizens.

First visit. It is a good idea to select a doctor while you are well, so you will not have to call on a stranger if you get sick. Having a complete physical is a good way for you and your doctor to get to know each other and to provide a review of your overall medical history and present physical condition. It may also identify some problems for which you are at particular risk.

Blood pressure check. No one disputes the value of detecting severe or even moderate high blood pressure before it causes any symptoms or trouble. Strokes and kidney failure *can* be prevented by adequate treatment of high blood pressure. Checking blood pressure is cheap and harmless. A must. How often? If your blood pressure is perfectly normal, every three or four years will probably do. There is controversy about how and if to treat the mild case—this decision has to be individualized.

Breast cancer check. Another test of proved value. Annual breast exam and mammography reduce deaths due to breast cancer. These tests do result in many biopsies of benign conditions and are expensive—but they increase the cure rate. Controversy exists about how often the test should be done and at what ages. There is general acceptance that women over fifty should have yearly exams; some argue for beginning screening earlier, but the data do not conclusively show that to be of value. Many experts recommend that women be trained in breast self-exam (BSE) but there is no data that proves its efficacy.

PAP smears. PAP smears detect cancer of the cervix before it causes symptoms and while (usually) easily cured. Although never scientifically "proved," this is generally accepted. There is some dispute about how often PAP smears should be done, with estimates varying from one to four years. All agree that women should start having PAP smears when they first become sexually active. PAP smears become less important in old age, and are probably not necessary after age seventy. Proper interpretation of a PAP smear requires skilled technicians who do not have an excessive work load. It wouldn't hurt to ask your doctor if he knows how reliable his laboratory is.

Cholesterol. Detecting and treating high cholesterol is definitely of benefit to the high-risk group—young or middle-aged men who smoke cigarettes and/or have a family history of heart attacks. Its value in patients over age seventy, and persons at low risk of heart disease (nonsmokers with normal blood pressure and a negative family history, especially women) is not proved.

All persons in the categories as noted should have these screening tests. The next group of tests include some about which the experts disagree. I recommend the ones listed below for my patients.

Colon cancer screening. Usually done only after age forty or even fifty, the stool test for occult blood and some form of colon visualization is commonly recommended. In recent years the availability of a flexible fiberoptic scope of 50 or 60 cm (about 3.5 feet) long has made a thorough examination of the rectum and colon possible with minimal risk and no more than moderate lower discomfort. Ideally, the test should be done two years in a row (to make sure no lesion is missed the first time) and then every three years.

Physical examination for certain early cancers. Examination of the skin, the mouth and throat, the lymph glands throughout the body, the thyroid gland in the neck, the testicles, the uterus and ovaries, and the prostate gland may, on occasion, detect an early and otherwise unnoticed cancer or precancerous condition. Most of these cancers become increasingly common as you age so you should be examined more frequently as you get older—every year after age fifty.

Electrocardiogram. An EKG is not much good as a screening test for heart disease, but it may be useful to have a base-line tracing for later comparison. Every person's EKG is a little different—almost like a fingerprint. Even some perfectly healthy people will have an "abnormal" EKG. If you should be one of those, and if you have suspicious but noncardiac chest pains, your EKG might lead to a wrong diagnosis of heart disease. But if a base-line tracing done in the past shows that there has been no change, it might be easier to arrive at the correct diagnosis. I try to get at least one base-line EKG in every regular patient's chart.

Osteoporosis prevention. Osteoporosis is very common in women after natural menopause and after surgical menopause caused by surgical removal of the ovaries. The bones become thin and fragile and may break after even minor injury. Osteoporosis can be prevented by taking estrogen hormone but estrogen can cause some discomfort and has some risks. Osteoporosis prevention is a controversial topic at present, and the decision about using estrogen ought to be arrived at after consultation with your doctor. Certain women are at higher risk than others; they are small-boned, fair-skinned, have a family history of osteoporosis, and smoke cigarettes. Such women probably should use estrogen at the time of menopause unless there is a compelling reason not to. Obese black women who don't smoke are at the other end of the spectrum—they are at much less risk.

9

MEDICAL MALPRACTICE
Carolyn Lavecchia, R.N., F.N.P., M.S., J.D.

Medical malpractice is not new to the legal system. Throughout the ages, physicians have been confronted with charges of malpractice. Although in ancient times the physician did not consider the possibility of a lawsuit, he practiced at great risk because he was considered an insurer of his care—that is, he guaranteed good results. Unlike today, the ancient world made no distinction between an unavoidable bad result and a bad result due to negligence. The Code of Hammurabi, enacted in approximately 2000 B.C., stated:

> If the surgeon has made a deep incision in the body of a free man and has caused the man's death, or has opened the caruncle in the eye and so destroys the man's eye, they shall cut off his forehands.

Fortunately—or unfortunately—a physician's failure to cure a slave or poor man resulted in lesser penalties.

One of the earliest recorded malpractice cases was in England in 1374, where a surgeon was sued for negligent treatment of a hand. Although the patient lost the case on a technicality, the court established the following early definition of malpractice applicable to doctors as well as blacksmiths, patients as well as horses:

> If a smith undertakes to cure a horse, and the horse is harmed by his negligence or failure to cure in a reasonable time, it is just that he should be held liable.

In the American legal system, patients have always had the right to sue their physicians for malpractice. In the first reported malpractice case in the

United States in 1794, a husband sued a doctor for the death of his wife, because of the doctor's negligence in performing an operation. The husband was awarded damages by the jury.

Over the next several decades, malpractice cases in the United States continued. In the mid-1800s, Abraham Lincoln unsuccessfully defended two doctors in a malpractice action. Indeed, it was during this time that the first "medical malpractice crisis" occurred, when physicians became concerned about the number of lawsuits being filed.

Following the Civil War, the crisis abated until the 1920s. By this time, insurance companies had begun providing coverage for physicians' negligence. Interestingly, in this period, another crisis occurred, during which some companies tripled their rates and others refused to write policies for physicians.

Ironically, the basic issues surrounding medical malpractice today are strikingly similar to the earlier days. While modern medicine is far more complex, with more scientific advances, new technology, and the development of physician specialization, medical malpractice actions and the medical malpractice crisis continue.

WHAT IS MEDICAL MALPRACTICE?

Usually when a physician is sued by a patient because of the physician's treatment, it is a suit for malpractice. Simply stated, malpractice is professional negligence. It is the failure of a physician to exercise the requisite degree of care, skill, and diligence, thereby resulting in harm to the patient.

Negligence is the legal theory you or any patient would most commonly use in a lawsuit against a physician.* In fact, negligence is the same legal theory employed in a lawsuit against the driver who negligently caused an auto accident. In order to be successful in a medical-negligence action, the plaintiff must prove four elements:

Duty. He or she must establish that the physician owed him a legal duty. In order for a duty to exist, there must be a physician-patient relationship.

Breach of duty. He must prove that the physician failed to comply with accepted professional standards.

Causation. He must establish a causal relationship between the physician's actions or omissions and the injury he suffered.

Damages. He must establish that he has suffered harm.

---
*The legal theory of negligence may also be used by patients in a lawsuit against other health-care providers, such as nurses, hospitals, pharmacists, and dentists. The same basic legal principles of negligence that are discussed in this chapter also apply to health-care providers other than physicians.

Duty

The physician-patient relationship usually arises voluntarily when you seek health care from a physician. Ordinarily, a physician has no duty to render services to anyone (unless he is employed at a governmental agency providing health services to the public). Once the physician undertakes to treat you as a patient, however, he then owes a duty of reasonable care and cannot abandon that care. This is true even where the physician has no face-to-face contact with you. For example, radiologists and physicians who work in laboratories often have no direct contact with patients, yet they owe them a legal duty nevertheless. The fact that a physician may render his services without charge also does not absolve him of his legal duty of care.

The duty created by the physician-patient relationship requires the physician to use such reasonable, ordinary care, skill, and diligence as a physician in the same general type of practice would ordinarily exercise in a similar situation. This duty is commonly referred to as the *standard of care*. By this definition, we can see that the physician is held to a standard of care defined by his own profession. It is important to note that standard of care is a duty of reasonable care and does not require the highest possible degree of care—only ordinary and reasonable care under the circumstances. A case of malpractice will exist only when the actions of your physician fall short of the accepted standards of his profession. Furthermore, your physician will not be held liable for a mere error of judgment. Unlike ancient times, today's physician is not an insurer of care. He has only a duty to use reasonable care and exercise his best judgment to effect a good result for you.

When a physician is a specialist, he is required to exercise the degree of skill, knowledge, and care which is ordinarily possessed by similar specialists, not that of a general practitioner. However, when a general practitioner or any physician undertakes your treatment, and your condition falls within a special field of medicine, he may be held to the standard of care for a specialist in that particular field of medicine. For example, if a general practitioner undertakes to treat a leg fracture, he may be held to the standard of care of an orthopedic surgeon.

A physician has a duty to obtain your consent to surgical procedures and other courses of treatment. In situations where the patient is a minor or is incompetent, a parent or guardian is usually required to give consent. Years ago this duty was nonexistent. Instead, the "doctor knows best" rule was in effect. Patients were considered incapable of understanding the complexities of medicine. But times have changed.

In addition to the duty to obtain your consent to treatment, your physician also has a duty to advise you of the nature of your illness and the possible risks of any proposed treatment, so you can make an informed decision concerning your available choices. This is usually referred to as *informed consent*. Explanations of your condition and the risks of proposed treatment should always be in terms you can understand. Your physician's duty to obtain consent and informed consent is based on your right, as the patient, to determine what shall be done to your own body.

There are two general exceptions to the duty to obtain informed consent. The first exception is in an emergency, where a patient is incapable of consenting and the risk of harm from failure to treat is greater than the risk of harm from the proposed treatment—typically when an auto-accident victim is brought into a hospital emergency room unconscious. The second exception is where the patient has a psychiatric condition that makes him fearful of any treatment. This situation is rare because of the increased recognition by the legal system of the patient's right to make informed decisions as to what happens to his body.

Breach of Duty

Your physician has a duty to practice with the degree of care ordinarily practiced by physicians in the same area of specialization. A violation of this duty—or breach, as it is called in legal jargon—occurs where the physician fails to meet this standard. Proof of the breach of the standard of care generally requires expert testimony. Usually you, as the plaintiff, will need an expert physician with similar education, training, and practice or area of specialization as your physician to testify that your doctor failed to meet the standard of care. Thus, a general practitioner or cardiologist will have difficulty testifying as to the standard of care for a neurosurgeon. Acts of omission as well as commission on the part of the physician may constitute a breach of the standard of care. Failure to order or perform diagnostic studies that most reasonable physicians would have done is an example of an omission; selection of an inappropriate course of treatment would be an example of a commission.

Because experts commonly disagree on the appropriate course of treatment for a given condition, it is imperative that a plaintiff-patient have an expert with good credentials. The plaintiff in a malpractice action has the burden of proof and has to establish by a preponderance (greater weight) of the evidence that the defendant doctor was negligent. In other words, the plaintiff has to show that the greater number of physicians in the same area of practice as the defendant doctor would not have acted as the defendant doctor did.

The standard of care is dependent upon the state of scientific knowledge and practice at the time of the alleged act of negligence, not at the time of trial. Hence, a physician will not be held to new scientific advances or today's standard of care for something that happened years before, as where a child sustains a birth injury due to medical malpractice and the action on his behalf is not brought until he is much older or has reached majority: The doctor's negligence must be proved within the context of medical knowledge at the time of the birth injury.

There are a few recognized exceptions to the expert testimony requirement. The most common example is where the physician's lack of care is obvious and easily comprehensible to the average lay person and not of a scientific or technical nature, as in the case where a surgeon leaves an instrument inside a patient during an operation. Most cases, however, do not fall within this exception.

In most cases, your physician has more than one option of treatment, any of which meet acceptable standards. It is not a breach of the standard of care if your physician chooses an option that is unsuccessful. The doctor only has a duty to use his or her best judgment and is not liable just because in exercising his good judgment the desired result is not achieved.

A physician may breach the duty of care by failure to obtain your consent for surgery or treatment. In cases where you do not consent to a specific surgery or treatment, your physician may be liable under the legal theories of assault and battery rather than negligence.*

Questions arise concerning what constitutes consent. As stated, except in an emergency or where you are unable to give consent, you must personally consent to the treatment. When you come to a physician's office seeking treatment and submit to a particular treatment, consent is usually implied. Usually upon admission to a hospital, you or a person legally qualified to give consent for you signs a general consent to treatment. For surgical procedures and treatment with a high degree of risk, such as the use of an experimental drug, you will usually be required to give a separate written consent.

Informed consent is more complex than consent. The primary issue surrounding informed consent is what information must be disclosed. Your physician must make sure that you fully understand the proposed treatment or surgical procedure and the associated risks. On the other hand, the physician has to exercise some discretion in explaining the risks so as not to alarm you unduly. You should ask questions, and if you do not understand what the physician is saying, you should ask him to explain it in simpler terms. Even though you may sign a consent form, if your signature is obtained without reasonable disclosure, then informed consent is not present. Generally, the information that must be disclosed is based upon what a reasonable physician

---

*Assault is defined as the act of placing a person in apprehension of harm. Battery is defined as the offensive touching of another without the consent or authorization of that person. Assault and battery are intentional torts. In a action against a physician for assault and battery for failure to obtain consent, it is not necessary that the physician have any hostile intent, only that he failed to obtain the patient's consent. An example of the application of these theories would be where you consented to surgery on your nose, but instead the surgeon removed your tonsils.

under similar facts and circumstances would disclose. Because this is a medical decision, expert testimony is required to establish a breach of the standard of care for failure to obtain informed consent.

Causation

To win a case of malpractice, the plaintiff must prove that the physician's acts or omissions legally (or proximately) caused the plaintiff's harm. Medical causation and legal causation are quite different. For medical causation the physician seeks to identify the most immediate cause or underlying causes and aspects of your problem.

Legal causation is more specific—whether a particular act or omission by the physician caused your injury. This means that the plaintiff has the burden of proving the physician's conduct is the cause which in a natural and continuing sequence, unbroken by any independent intervening cause, produces injury. Although causation may be proved by direct or circumstantial evidence, because of the technical complexity of the subject matter, expert testimony is usually required. To prove proximate cause, a plaintiff does not have to establish with absolute certainty that a specific act or failure to act by the physician caused the injury; however, a plaintiff has to show to a reasonable degree of probability that the injury was caused by the physician's conduct.

Proving proximate cause often presents the most difficult aspect of proving a medical malpractice case. In some instances, a patient may have suffered a serious injury, such as the loss of a limb or even death. Although the physician may have breached the standard of care, proving that this breach was the cause of the bad result—rather than another cause, such as the natural course or complications of the patient's illness or injury—can in complex cases be compared to the difficulty of unscrambling an egg.

Damages

The final element that has to be proved in a negligence action against a physician is damages. This is simply the harm or injury suffered by the patient due to the negligence of a physician. The law recognizes three general areas of damages: general damages, special damages, and punitive damages.

General damages are those damages which necessarily result from the injury, such as emotional distress, pain, and suffering. *Special damages* are the actual but not the necessary result of the injury suffered. Typical special damages are past and future medical and hospital expenses, past and future loss of income, loss of earning capacity, and funeral expenses in the case of a death. The purpose of general and special damages is to compensate the injured party. *Punitive* or *exemplary damages* are damages to punish a defendant for outrageous conduct and to deter such conduct in the future.

Thus, acts of negligence alone are insufficient as a basis for punitive damages.

Simple negligence on the part of a physician is a failure to exercise reasonable or ordinary care. However serious the injury suffered as a result, (even death), this does not mean that simple negligence is a case for punitive damages; for the purposes of punitive damages, *the conduct of the physician* is the issue not *the injury*. This conduct has to be outrageous, reckless, willful, wanton, or in conscious disregard for the rights or safety of others. Thus, punitive damages are rarely awarded in medical malpractice actions.

The Patient's Duty

You, as a patient, also have legal duty. You are required to conform to the same standard of conduct as would a reasonable person of under similar circumstances. Even though your physician is found to be negligent and would otherwise be liable, you may be denied recovery if you failed to act in a reasonable manner yourself. This is called contributory negligence, and in some states may bar any recovery. For example, if you fail to follow your doctor's treatment plan, and this failure causes you injury, then you will likely be found contributorily negligent, since most reasonable patients would follow the instructions of their physicians. Because of the harshness of this rule, other states have what is termed comparative negligence. Under the comparative-negligence doctrine, there is an apportionment of damages based upon the plaintiff's degree of fault.

TYPES OF MEDICAL MALPRACTICE CASES

Most medical malpractice actions can be placed in the following categories:

Diagnostic errors. A situation in which a physician may be found negligent for a diagnostic error would be the failure to obtain a specific diagnostic test when presented with certain signs and symptoms. For example, a fifty-year-old male who comes to an emergency-room physician with the classic signs and symptoms of a heart attack. If this patient is sent out of the emergency room by the physician without having obtained an electrocardiogram and the patient dies shortly afterward of a heart attack, the physician will likely be found negligent. Although an electrocardiogram may not have shown the patient was suffering a heart attack, more likely than not it would, and most emergency-room physicians would have obtained one.

Just because a physician makes an incorrect diagnosis does not necessarily mean he is negligent. The critical issue is whether the physician employed the reasonable care and skill of a general practitioner or specialist under like circumstances.

Surgical procedures. Although there is some risk associated with most surgical procedures, if your surgeon fails to take the necessary precautions to prevent the occurrence of these risks, then he may be liable for malpractice. For example, if a surgeon fails to provide a sufficient quantity of blood to control hemorrhage during the surgery or fails to recognize post-operative hemorrhage, which is a recognized risk of most major surgeries, he may be liable if the patient suffers a resulting injury.

Another common source of liability arising out of surgical procedures is foreign bodies, such as gauze sponges, instruments, or drainage tubes, being left in the patient. In most cases, this does not meet acceptable standards. Another situation for which patients often consult an attorney is the inadvertent stitching or cutting of a blood vessel, nerve, or something in the operative area. Surprisingly, in most cases this is not due to negligence, but occurs because of anatomical variations or the difficulty of discerning the vessel, etc. As long as the surgeon takes appropriate steps to anticipate this risk, then the standard of care is not violated. However, failure to recognize this complication in a timely manner may result in negligence.

Anesthesia. There are a growing number of cases of anesthesia mishaps. These cases usually arise out of problems with the anesthetic drugs, ventilation, oxygenation, and monitoring of the patient's vital signs and condition for complications. Use of the wrong drug, the incorrect drug dose, or failure to use a drug may be grounds for negligence. Providing adequate oxygenation for a patient is a critical role for the anesthesiologist. For example, if the breathing tube is placed in the esophagus instead of the trachea, then the oxygen will go into the stomach and not the lungs. Inadvertent placement of the tube can happen in the best of hands, but failure to recognize and correct this problem is usually inexcusable. Failure of the anesthesiologist to keep a continuous monitor on the patient's vital signs, such as the blood pressure, pulse, respiration, and temperature in the operating room and the recovery room is also a source of liability in malpractice actions involving anesthesia mishaps.

Treatment errors. Treatment errors that can result in malpractice actions span all areas of medical practice. They range from inadequate treatment, such as failure to hospitalize or treat appropriately a bacterial infection, to prescribing excessive narcotics or some nonnarcotic drugs, which cause the patient to become addicted.

Drug errors. The huge volume of drugs on the market and the growing number of patients on multiple prescriptions and nonprescription drugs create an increased risk of errors by physicians and patients. Errors can range from an incorrect dose to the wrong drug.

Emergencies. Most states have Good Samaritan statutes that provide some protection for physicians who render emergency care—immunity from liability for civil damages as long as there is no gross negligence or willful or wanton conduct. This immunity is usually inapplicable to the physician in emergency rooms, where the patient is taken following an accident or some other emergency.

Failure to obtain consultation. With the increasing specialization and subspecialization in medicine, in most cases where a patient is seriously ill, consultation with medical specialists is usually the standard. If the patient's condition is beyond the education and training or area of practice of the physician, the physician may be negligent if he fails to consult with the appropriate specialists, and the patient suffers harm.

Birth injuries. In recent years, there has been a growing number of malpractice actions for birth injuries, the most common being neurological or brain injury. These injuries range from a learning disorder to severe brain damage and may result from the physician's failure to recognize signs of fetal distress. The upshot is neurological damage for the infant and a malpractice action against the physician.

Psychiatric Conditions. There is a developing trend of malpractice actions against psychiatrists—for example, in cases where a patient commits suicide or harms a third party. Where most reasonable psychiatrists would have known that the patient posed a risk for harm to himself and others, failure of the psychiatrist to take appropriate steps to prevent such foreseeable harm may result in the psychiatrist being found negligent.

IN THERE A CASE?

Usually the question of medical malpractice arises only when medical treatment of a patient or family member suffers an unsatisfactory outcome. But it cannot be overemphasized that not every bad outcome is the result of negligence. Indeed, most bad results are simply the natural course of an illness or its complications or of a severe injury, not malpractice. Some bad outcomes, however, should rouse your suspicions. For example, when a young, otherwise healthy person, with what appears to be a relatively minor illness, suffers serious complications or even death, you should consider the possibility of malpractice. Another example would be when a relatively healthy person undergoes a surgical procedure with little known risk and subsequently has serious complications or dies. Whenever a physician expresses uneasiness about the care and treatment rendered by another physician, you should be concerned that malpractice may have occurred.

In most instances, whenever you have questions about your treatment or proposed treatment, you should first talk with your physician. Most physicians will be open and forthright and try to answer your questions as best they can. Most likely your concerns will be alleviated. If a communication problem exists between you and your physician, such a discussion may be difficult for both of you. If you suspect that information is being withheld from you, you are unlikely to be satisfied with the physician's replies and may look elsewhere for an explanation.

At some point you may consider consulting an attorney. Before doing so, you should first ask yourself: What harm have I suffered? Not infrequently patients are upset because of a personality clash with the physician or surgeon. The courts do not offer any relief where the harm is merely hurt feelings or the result of bad bedside manners. Generally there must be some substantial physical or economic harm.

Medical malpractice cases are as complex for the attorney as the practice of medicine is itself. The legal principles are relatively simple, but determining whether or not there is a case of medical malpractice is not so simple. Therefore, you will be wise to consult an attorney who is experienced in the area of medical malpractice or other types of personal injury.

If you do not know such an attorney or a law firm that meets this criterion, you should ask an attorney in whom you have confidence to refer you. Or consult the local bar association and request the names of several attorneys whose practice is in the area of medical malpractice or personal injury.

Do not delay. All states have statutes that set forth a specified period of time in which a lawsuit must be brought—statutes of limitations. If your suit is not commenced within the required period of time, no matter how meritorious your claim or how great your injury, it will usually be dismissed. Statutes of limitations vary from one to five years, depending on the state. In some instances, such as the case of a minor, the statute of limitations may not begin to run until the patient reaches the age of majority. In some instances, it may not begin to run until the course of treatment by the negligent physician ends. Again, these rules vary from state to state. In order to protect your rights, consult an attorney as soon as possible.

Even an attorney experienced in medical malpractice cases is unlikely to be able to advise you immediately whether you have or don't have a case. He probably will need to review your medical records and to confer with an expert physician before telling you whether you should proceed.

Most attorneys will provide you with an initial consultation free of charge. Charges thereafter may vary. Some attorneys may charge a fee to evaluate whether you have a case, while others may not. If an attorney undertakes to represent you in a malpractice action, the case will usually be on the basis of a contingency fee—that is, the attorney receives a percentage of the amount you recover. If you fail to recover any damages, through either an out-of-court settlement or a verdict, then the attorney receives no compensation at all for his legal services. The reason for contingency fee is that most people are unable to retain an attorney at an hourly rate. This preparation time can be quite lengthy, because of the complexity of most medical malpractice cases. Without a contingency-fee arrangement, many injured persons would be unable to afford legal assistance at all and would therefore be unable to obtain compensation for their injury. If you prefer, you can retain an attorney on an hourly rate. You should inquire as to the attorney's charges for consultation and investigation of your case during your initial contact with him. All attorneys are required to give you this information.

You should also be aware that expenses will be incurred in the investigation of your potential case. The major cost items are copying charges for your medical records and the fees to have an expert physician or other health-care provider reviewing those records. Most expert physicians charge at least $100 per hour to review medical records and confer with an attorney. If it becomes necessary to obtain an evaluation from more than one expert and if the medical records are voluminous, these expenses can easily mount up. Investigation costs may range from several hundred dollars to several thousand, depending on the case and whether the attorney has an initial investigation fee. Importantly, whether you ultimately have a case of malpractice or not, you, the client, are responsible for paying bills incurred either in the investigation of your case or in the actual litigation. This is a requirement of the Legal Code of Ethics of the American Bar Association. This requirement does not preclude your attorney from advancing costs; however, ultimately you must pay for them. In your initial meeting with our attorney, you should discuss estimated costs, since these vary from case to case, and you need to know as early as possible what the action is going to cost you.

If an attorney declines to take your case, it may be for several reasons. He may have a conflict of interest—perhaps represents or has represented the potential defendant doctor. Or the case may have little, if any, likelihood of success, usually because of an inability to prove one or more of the required elements of duty, breach of duty, causation, and damages. In this case, listen very carefully to the attorney's explanation of why your case is weak, particularly if an objective physician has reviewed the records. If you are dissatisfied with this explanation, you may wish to consult another attorney.

Because of the many advances in medical science, Americans generally have a high expectation of health care. When a patient suffers a bad outcome, he or his family often conclude that the health-care provider must be at fault. Often their aroused emotions interfere with calm and rational thought, and as a result, it is often difficult for them to accept the fact that the physician's care and treatment were not below the standard of care, that they did not cause the harm suffered.

In legal jargon, a case that is not valid is called frivolous or without merit. If your case lacks merit, it is likely that it will be dismissed at some point during the proceedings, usually without ever reaching the trial stage. Indeed, the federal courts have a rule that provides for sanctions or a fine if frivolous cases are commenced. States are now beginning to enact similar provisions. Thus, you are unlikely to find an attorney to commence any action on your behalf unless your case has merit.

Every American has the right to represent himself in court. As a practical matter, however, without the training and resources of an experienced malpractice lawyer, a layman has little chance of success. A plaintiff representing himself would be fortunate to avoid the imposition of sanctions.

You should realize that a lawsuit for malpractice is emotionally demanding for a patient, his family, the physician, and other health-care providers. Although you may be upset or angry at your physician, filing a medical malpractice case is not the appropriate outlet for those emotions. Indeed, pursuing a nonmeritorious case against your physician—or anyone else, for that matter—will only lead to further emotional upset and financial loss.

If an attorney concludes that you have a meritorious case, he will commence action on your behalf. The procedure varies from state to state. In some states your case may be filed directly in court; in others it may be heard first by a medical malpractice review panel, which was created as an arbitration or mediation procedure to weed out nonmeritorious claims and encourage prompt settlement of valid claims. In some states, panels are mandatory, while in other states they are optional. In those states with review panels, you still have the right to proceed to court after the panel decision, whether it was favorable or unfavorable to you.

Ordinarily your case is filed in a state trial court, but it may be filed in federal court if the defendant physician or other health-care provider is an employee of the federal government or armed forces, or if you and your doctor are not residents of the same state or if one of you is not a citizen of the United States.

Medical malpractice cases are civil actions, not criminal. In a civil action the procedural rules and requirements are quite different from those in a criminal prosecution, and there is no government prosecutor. The parties, or two sides to the lawsuit, are you, the plaintiff, and the doctor (or doctors or hospital), the defendant.

Once your case has been filed, information will be exchanged between the plaintiff and defendant. This will be done through written questions to be answered under oath, and through the exchange of documents and depositions. In a complex case, which most medical malpractice cases are, you, the defendant doctor, and other health-care providers will usually be required to give a deposition. A deposition is where a potential witness at trial is questioned under oath by counsel to determine what the witness' testimony will likely be at trial. Experts, too, may be required either to produce a written report or to give a deposition. This pretrial exchange of information is called discovery, and its purpose is to allow each party to discover what testimony the opponent will use at trial. Modern-day trials simply do not have the Perry Mason type of suspense and surprise, because discovery permits each party the opportunity to have a general idea what the testimony of his opponent's witnesses will be.

If your case gets to court, the trial will usually last anywhere from a day to several weeks, depending upon the number of witnesses and the complexity of your case. In most instances you will have a jury trial, although in a few instances your case may be heard only by a judge. Most plaintiffs request a jury trial whenever possible. The jury decides all issues of fact, whereas the judge decides the legal issues and instructs the jury as to what law the jury must apply in deciding the facts. In a case where there is no jury, the judge decides both issues of law and fact.

After the final verdict is reached and judgment is entered, either party may appeal that decision. Unlike criminal proceedings, civil actions may not have an automatic right of appeal. The appeals court may decide whether it will even consider the case. If an appeal is granted, the appeals court usually does not redecide the facts, but considers only erroneous legal rulings by the trial judge. For example, if the judge did not allow your attorney to introduce some important evidence that affected the outcome of the case, the appellate court may reverse all or part of the decision and order a new trial. Oftentimes an appeals court may affirm the trial-court decision, thus ending the case. If your case is in state court, the appeal is only to the state appeals court, usually the highest court in the state such as the state supreme court. For a case in state court, there is really no appeal to any federal court. If, however, your case was filed and tried in a federal trial court, it may then be appealed to the appropriate federal circuit court.

After the appeal process is exhausted (or if neither party appeals the trial-court decision), then your case is final. The process from the filing of the lawsuit to trial may take several years in states where court dockets are busy, and lawsuits move slowly. If your case is then appealed, this could take another several years. For an injured person in need of compensation to provide for medical expenses, economic support, and other needs, it may be a long time before any of the much-needed compensation reaches him. Although this delay is frequently criticized, it is a major problem confronting any person injured by the negligence of another. Unfortunately, this delay occurs with other civil actions as well.

An out-of-court settlement may occur at any time during the legal proceedings. Indeed, it may even occur before any lawsuit is filed. The major advantage of an out-of-court settlement for an injured plaintiff is that it represents guaranteed compensation to an injured person without having to go through the lengthy litigation process. Settlements may also be structured, with the plaintiff receiving a periodic payment, on a monthly or yearly basis, as opposed to receiving all of the money in one lump sum. The advantage of structured settlements is that the injured person is guaranteed an income on a periodic basis, and this usually results in his receiving more money in the long run. The advantages for a defendant or a defendant's insurance company is that the money can be invested to offset the greater amount to be paid out long-term.

INSURANCE CRISIS OR MEDICAL MALPRACTICE CRISIS?

Since the mid-1970s, costs of liability insurance premiums for physicians and other health-care providers have increased drastically. Initially, lawyers, physicians, and other health-care providers and even patients were blamed for this occurrence. Liability-insurance carriers declared that the increased premium costs were necessary to offset the dramatic increase in the number of malpractice actions being filed and the increasingly higher jury verdicts being awarded plaintiffs.

Concomitantly, health-care costs have escalated as well, also attributed to an increased number of malpractice lawsuits. It was claimed that physicians were ordering too many unnecessary diagnostic studies, "defensive medicine," because of their fear of lawsuits. The consumer or the patient was also accused of driving up the costs of health care and liability insurance premiums by being too litigious.

As a result, some physicians who have never been sued for medical malpractice have nonetheless seen their rates more than quadruple. Some physicians have experienced difficulty in affording and even obtaining liability coverage. In some areas, patients have been unable to obtain certain types of health care, particularly obstetrical.

Because of these events, some state legislatures have enacted legislation placing restrictions on the amount of damages a plaintiff can recover in a medical malpractice action. Such measures include statutory restrictions or a "cap" on the total amount any plaintiff may recover, regardless of the severity of the injury. For example, in some states, even if a plaintiff is able to prove that he has experienced huge medical expenses in the past and will incur a large amount in future, the cap may severely restrict the amount he may recover. Some states have placed limits on the amount an injured person may recover for pain and suffering and punitive damages. As a result, the less severely injured person may be fairly and reasonably compensated, but the severely injured one must suffer not only from his severe injury but from inadequate compensation. Not surprisingly, these laws have been challenged as unconstitutional and have indeed been overturned in some states. However, in other states they are still in existence and must be reckoned with by a patient injured as the result of medical malpractice.

Interestingly, in the 1980s, the name has changed from "medical malpractice crisis" to "insurance crisis." Members of the legal profession have commenced an investigation into the causes of this crisis, and these investigations suggest that the problem is not caused by litigious society, an increased number of malpractice actions, or high jury verdicts, but by problems in the insurance industry and the way it had invested its money. Consequently, states are taking a harsh look at the industry and are imposing stricter regulations on liability-insurance carriers, including closer scrutiny of rate increases and stricter reporting requirements. Just recently, a lawsuit was filed in federal court by some states' attorneys general against some of the major liability-insurance carriers alleging that they conspired to limit commercial liability coverage and to charge excessive prices. Private class-action lawsuits with similar allegations have also been filed. Although it may be some time before the facts are fully known, we will probably survive another medical malpractice crisis, if indeed there was one.

In conclusion, medical care has grown tremendously in complexity since ancient times, yet human error has not been eliminated and medical malpractice lawsuits have steadily increased over the years. While most physicians are dedicated to the practice of medicine, and their practice is well within the standards of their profession, medical negligence does occur, and our American legal system provides a means for compensation for the person injured by the negligence of the physician. Indirectly, this legal right benefits society with an improvement in the quality of health care. It is in society's interest that the legal system continues to allow meritorious claims for malpractice.

BIBLIOGRAPHY

Introduction
1. Abraham Flexner, *The Flexner Report*. Reprint: Washington, D.C.: Science and Health Publications, 1960.
2. Jacob A. Bigelow, *A Discourse on Self-Limited Disease*. Boston: Ticknor & Fields, 1854.

Chapter 1
1. A.N. Marquis Co., *Directory of Medical Specialists*, 22d ed., 1985.

Chapter 2
1. Joseph J. Falkson, "HMOs and the Politics of Health System Reform." *American Hospital Association,* Chicago, Illinois, 1980.
2. R. J. Arnold, L. W. Debrock, J. W. Pollard, "Do HMOs Produce Specific Services More Efficiently?" *Inquiry*, Fall 1984, 21(3):243–53.
3. M. J. Long, "An integrated theory of provider behavior in Health Maintenance Organizations." *Journal of Community Health*: Winter 1982, 8(2):119–29.
4. J. P. LoGerfo, R. A. Efird, P. K. Diehr, "Rates of surgical care in prepaid group practices and the independent setting: what are the reasons for the differences? *Medical Care*, January 1979, 17(1):1–10.
5. Beeck M. Jackson, J. H. Kleinman, "Evidence for self-selection among health maintenance organization enrollees." *Journal of American Medical Association*, 1983 November 25; 250(20):2826–9.
6. Richard McNeil, Jr., and Robert E. Schlenker, "HMOs, Competition and Government." *Milbank Memorial Fund Quarterly*, Spring 1975: 1195–1224.
7. S. E. Berki, Marie Ashcraft, "HMO enrollment: Who joins what and why: A review of the literature." *Milbank Memorial Fund Quarterly*, 1980, 58(4):588–632.
8. Steven A. Schroeder and Molla S. Donaldson, "The feasibility of an outcome approach to quality assurance—a report from one HMO." *Medical Care*, 1976, 14(1):49–56.
9. J. K. Barr, M. K. Steinberg, "A physician role typology: colleague and client dependence in an HMO." *Social Science Medicine*, 1985, 20(3):253–261.

10. Milton I. Roemer, William Shonick, "HMO performance: the recent evidence." *Milbank Memorial Fund Quarterly*, Summer 1973: 278.
11. James P. LoGerfo, Eric Larson, William C. Richardson, "Assessing the quality of care for urinary tract infection in office practice." *Medical Care*, 1978, 16(56):488–495.
12. James P. LoGerfo, "Organizational and financial influences on patterns of surgical care." *Surgical Clinics of North America*, 1982, 62(4):677–684.
13. Charles H. Wright, T. Hershel Gardin, Carla L. Wright, "Obstetric care in a health maintenance organization and a private fee-for-service practice: a comparative analysis." *American Journal of Obstetrics and Gynecology*, 1984, 149(8):848–856.
14. Elizabeth M. Sloss, Emmett B. Keeler, Robert H. Brook et al., "Effect of a health maintenance organization on physiologic health—results from a randomized study." *Annals of Internal Medicine*, 1987, 106:130–138.
15. Peter Boland, ed. *The New Healthcare Market—A Guide to PPOs for Purchasers, Payors and Providers.* Homewood, IL: Dow Jones-Irwin, 1985.
16. Mayer, Thomas R., and Gloria Gilbert, *The Health Insurance Alternative—A Complete Guide to Health Maintenance Organizations.* New York: Putnam, 1984.
17. Associated Press wires, April 7, 1987.
18. Muriel Gillick, "The impact of health maintenance organizations on geriatric care." *Annals of Internal Medicine*, 1987, 106:139–143.

Chapter 3

1. J. W. Frank, "Occult-blood screening for colorectal carcinoma: the risks." *American Journal of Preventive Medicine*, 1985, 1(4):25–32.
2. W. Einthoven, "Die galvonometrische Registrierung des menschlichen Elektrocardiogramms." *Pflegers Archiv*, 1903, 99:472–480.

Chapter 4

1. Peter Temin, *Taking Your Medicine.* Cambridge, Mass: Harvard University Press, 1980.
2. Brian L. Storm, "Generic drug substitution revisited." *New England Journal of Medicine*, 1987, 316:1456–1462.
3. Neil J. Facchinetti, Michael W. Dickson, "Access to generic drugs in the 1950's: the politics of a social problem." *American Journal of Public Health*, 1982, 72:468–475.
4. D. S. Freestone, "Formulation and therapeutic efficacy of drugs used in clinical trials." *Lancet*, 1969, 2:98–99.
5. Leroy L. Schwartz, "The debate over substitution policy." *American Journal of Medicine*, 1985, 79 (Suppl. 2B):38–44.
6. D. C. Brater, W. A. Pettinger, "The generic prescribing issue." *Annals of Internal Medicine*, 1980, 92:426–427.
7. B. S. Bloom, D. J. Wierz, M. V. Pauly, "Cost and price of comparable branded and generic pharmaceuticals." *Journal of the American Medical Association*, 1986, 256:2523–2530.
8. L. Lasagna, "The economics of generic prescribing: winners and losers." *Journal of the American Medical Association*, 1986, 256:2566.

9. Robert J. Bolger, "Cost and price of comparable branded and generic pharmaceuticals." *Journal of the American Medical Association*, 1987, 257:2435–2438.
10. J. E. Goyan, "Letter to the editor." *Journal of the American Medical Association*, 1987, 257:2436.

Chapter 5

1. Lubin, L. F., *Medical Management of the Surgical Patient*. Boston: Butterworths, 1988.
2. Goldman, Lee, "Cardiac risks and complications of noncardiac surgery," *Annals of Internal Medicine*,98 (1983):504–13.
3. Psulka, P. S., et al., "The risks of surgery in obese patients," *Annals of Internal Medicine*, 104 (1983):540–46.
4. Moosa, A. R., et al., "Surgical complications," in D. C. Sabiston, ed., *Textbook of Surgery*, (Philadelphia: W. B. Saunders, 1986.
4a. Warner, M.D. et al., "Role of Preoperative cessation of smoking," Mayo Clinic Proceedings, (1989) 64(6):607–744.
5. Colombo, M., et al., "A multicenter, prospective study of post-transfusion hepatitis in Milan," *Hepatology*, (1987) 7(4):709–12.
6. Rutkow, I. M. "Unnecessary surgery: what is it?" *Surgical Clinics of North America*, (1982) 62 (4):613–25.
7. Grabova, T. B., et al., "Results of a second-opinion program for coronary artery bypass graft surgery," *Journal of the American Medical Association*, (1987) 258 (12):1611–1614.

Chapter 6

1. Marc A. Schuckit, "Genetics and the risk for alcoholism," *Journal of the American Medical Association*, 1985, 254:18, 2614.
2. Harvey B. Milkman and Howard J. Shaffer, *The Addictions*. Lexington, Mass.: Lexington Books, 1985.
3. Vernon E. Johnson, *I'll Quit Tomorrow*, San Francisco: Harper & Row, 1980.

Additional Suggested Reading

Alcoholics Anonymous, 3d ed., Alcoholics Anonymous World Services, Inc., New York: 1976.

Jean Kenney and Gwen Leaton, *Loosening the Grip*. St. Louis: C.V. Mosby Co., 1983.

Narcotics Anonymous. World Service Office, Inc., Van Nuys, California: 1984.

Richard Seymour and David E. Smith, *Guide to Psychoactive Drugs*. Harrington Park Press, Inc., New York: 1987.

Twelve Steps and Twelve Traditions. Alcoholics Anonymous World Services Inc., New York: 1978.

Janet G. Woititz, *Adult Children of Alcoholics*. Health Communications, Inc., Panpano Beach, Florida: 1983.

Chapter 7

1. E. M. Hamilton and S. Gropper, *The Biochemistry of Human Nutrition*. St. Paul, Minn.: West Publishing Company, 1987.

2. R. Pike and M. Brown, *Nutrition: An Integrated Approach*. 2nd ed., New York: John Wiley and Sons, 1975.
3. Joseph F. Califano, "American's health care revolution: health promotion and disease prevention." *Journal of the American Dietetic Association*, 1987, (IV):437–440.
4. The National Heart, Lung and Blood Institute, "Cholesterol treatment recommendations for adults: highlights of 1987 report." Oral presentation by the National Cholesterol Education Program Adult Treatment Panel on October 5, 1987.
5. M. Brown and J. Goldstein, "A receptor-mediated pathway for cholesterol homeostasis." *Science*, 1986, 232:34–47.
6. Proctor and Gamble research study, "Dietary fat in nutrition and cardiovascular health." 1987.
7. "The clinical role of fiber." Unpublished proceedings of symposium held at Toronto, Canada, February, 1985.
8. R. L. Atkinson, "Treatment strategies for hyperlipidemia." Paper presented at the Virginia Dietetic Association Fall Conference held at Williamsburg, Virginia, November 12–13, 1987.
9. J. Slavin, "Dietary fiber: classification, chemical analyses and food sources." *Journal of the American Dietetic Association*, 1987, 87(IX):1164–1171.
10. "All fiber is not created equal; colon cancer controversy." *Environmental Nutrition*, 1986, 9 (x).
11. "The fallacies of taking supplements." *Tufts University Diet and Nutrition Letter*, 1987, 5 (v).
12. "Tracing the facts about trace minerals." *Tufts University Diet and Nutrition Letter*. 1987, 5 (I).
13. "Vitamin B_6 toxicity and premenstrual syndrome." *Tufts University Diet and Nutrition Letter*, 1986, 3 (XII).
14. Recommended Dietary Allowance, The National Research Council, National Academy of Sciences, Washington, D.C., 1980.
15. "Zinc supplements: how much is too much?" *Tufts University Diet and Nutrition Letter*, 1985, 2 (XI).
16. National Institutes of Health Consensus Development Conference Statement, "Health implications of obesity." Washington, D.C.: U.S. government Printing Office, 1985m, 5 (IX).
17. G. Kolata, "Weight regulation may start in our cells, not psyches." *Smithsonian Magazine*, 1986, 16:91–97.
18. T. Morck, R. Atkinson, J. Foreyt et al., "Obesity: causes, consequences, and cures." Unpublished presentation at 4th Eastern Virginia Nutrition Conference. Williamsburg, Virginia, April 25–26, 1986.
19. National Dairy Council, *Weight management: A summary of current theory and practice*. Rosemont, Illinois, 1985.
20. WGBH Education Foundation, "Fat chance in a thin world." *NOVA*, No. 1007, 1983.
21. C. Bailey, *Fit or Fat*. Boston, Mass.: Houghton Mifflin Company, 1978.
22. "Eating disorders: how to detect the symptoms, where to go for help." *Environment Nutrition*, 1987, 10 (XI).
23. K. Brownell, "A program for managing obesity." *Dietetic Currents*. 1986, 13 (III).

Chapter 8
1. S. B. Hulley, J. B. Wyngaarden, ed., "Principles of preventive medicine." *Cecil Textbook of Medicine*. Philadelphia: W. B. Saunders, 1988.
2. S. B. Hulley, J. B. Wyngaarden, ed., "Control of unintended injuries and those due to violence." *Cecil Textbook of Medicine*, Philadelphia: W. B. Saunders, 1988.
3. F. R. Willis, ed., "Health implications of obesity—National Institutes of Health Consensus Development Conference Statement." *Annals of Internal Medicine*, 1985, 103 (6 pt 2):1073–1077.
4. E. L. Barrett-Conner, "Obesity, atherosclerosis and coronary artery disease." *Annals of Internal Medicine*, 1985, 103 (6 pt 2):1010–1019.
5. Committee on Immunization, Council, of Medical Societies, "Guide for adult immunization." *American College of Physicians*, Philadelphia, 1985.

Chapter 9
Suggested Reading
David Ghitelman, *The Natural History of Malpractice M.D.*, April 1987:59–81.

Harry A. Gair and Robert Conason, John Herbert Tovey, ed., *The Trial of a Negligence Action*. New York: Practising Law Institute, 1969.

Charles Kramer, *Medical Malpractice*. New York: Practising Law Institute, 1976.

James Walker Smith, *Hospital Liability*. New York: Law Journal Seminars-Press, 1985.

David W. Louisell and Harold Williams, *Medical Malpractice*, Vols. I and II. New York: Matthew Bender & Co., Inc. 1988.

INDEX

ACE inhibitors, 92
Accidents, 182
Activase, 101
Acyclovir, 91
Addiction, 145–52, 181, 195
  defined, 144
  to depressants, 140
  to painkillers, 90, 95
Adrenal gland, 19, 68, 73, 85, 96
Adrenalin (epinephrine), 77
Aerobics formula, 182–83
Aesculapius (Asclepius), 106
Age
  and surgical risk, 115, 116, 117
  and weight, 171
AIDS, 58, 59, 74, 99, 101, 144, 181
  blood transfusions and, 125
  testing for, 61
Ailments, coexisting
  and surgical risk, 115, 116–17
Alanon, 151, 152
Alateen, 151
Alcohol, 137–38, 139, 147, 181
  as depressant, 139–42
  and emergency surgery, 118–19
Alcoholics, 152, 164
Alcoholics Anonymous, 149–50
Alcoholism, 74, 98, 138, 148, 181
  as disease, 145
  treatment of, 148–50
Allergic reactions, 62, 76–78, 81, 144
Allergies, 17, 34, 96
Allergy medications, 95
Allopurinol, 97
Alzheimer's disease, 23, 74, 138
Amino acids, 154, 155, 163, 166
Ammonia, 141

Analgesics, 76
Anaphylaxis, 77
Anatomy, 106, 107, 108
Anemia, 20, 68, 97, 115, 167–68
Anesthesia, 108, 110, 121, 122, 136
  adverse reaction to, 78
  malpractice cases over, 195
  risks with, 115
Anesthesiology, 17, 19, 25, 117, 119, 120
Aneurism, 129, 132
Angina, 92, 114, 117, 143
Angiograms, 19, 63, 71, 72, 73
Anorexia nervosa, 174
Antacids, 84, 93
Antiarrhythmic drugs, 92–93
Antibiotics, 2, 3, 75, 76, 79, 81, 84, 91–92, 121, 122, 165
  allergic reaction to, 77, 78
  and kidney failure, 122
  new, 20, 101
  in prevention of infection, 117
  in surgery, 133
Antibodies, 70–71, 73, 98–99, 100
  and allergic reactions, 77
  proteins as, 155
Antibody tests, 68, 70
Anticonvulsants, 104
Antidepressants, 79, 94, 104
Antiepileptic drugs, 93
Antihistamines, 79, 90, 94, 95
Antihypertensives, 81, 92, 98, 101–2
Antipsychotic drugs, 94, 103
Antisepsis, 108, 109, 136
Antispasmodic drugs, 93
Arterial blockage, 132
Arthritis, 69, 90, 96, 113–14, 127, 129
  causes of, 20

Index

Arthroscopic surgery, 22, 67, 133
Artificial joints, 22
Artificial kidney, 20, 122
Asepsis, 109
Aspirin, 78, 95
Asthma, 17, 19, 72, 82, 90, 116, 121, 143
Asthma medications, 95–96
Atherosclerosis, 157–58, 183
Atrovent, 96
AZT, 91

Bacteria, 20, 69, 70, 91, 108, 158, 184, 187
  discovery of, 2
  intestinal, 165
Bacterial infections, 144
Balloon angioplasty, 19, 115, 130, 132
Barber surgeons, 106, 108
Barium enema, 62, 72
Barium X rays, 62, 71, 72
Benzodiazepams, 90, 94, 140
Beta agonists, 95–96
Beta blockers, 92, 93
Beta-carotene, 164
Bigelow, Jacob, 2
Bilirubin, 141
Biopsy, 58, 66, 70, 74, 134, 186
Birth-control pills, 87–88, 96, 122
Birth injuries, defects, 138, 192, 196
Bladder, 25, 67, 73, 123
Bleeding, 67, 74, 122, 195
Bleeding treatment, 2
Blood, 20, 111
  in stool, 60, 72, 187
  in urine, 67, 73
Blood-cholesterol measurement, 158–59, 164
Blood clots, 65, 101, 117, 132
  in leg veins, 121–22, 184
  in lungs, 19, 72
Blood fats, 19, 182
Blood-gas test, 72
Blood poisoning, 108, 144
Blood pressure, 92, 122, 141, 168, 186
  see also Hypertension
Blood pressure medications, 79, 90–91, 117
Blood sugar, 57, 61, 81, 97, 116
Blood tests, 68–69, 74
Blood thinners, 79, 81, 117, 122
Blood transfusions, 2, 108, 110–112, 128, 136
  autologous, 126, 131
  and surgical complications, 125–26
Blood type, typing, 112, 125
Blood vessels, surgery on, 130
Blundell, James, 111–112
Body chemistry, 78, 170–71

Body fluids, 69
Body specimens, 69–70
Boland, Peter, 42
Bone marrow, 20, 76, 141
Bone scan, 65
Brain, 63, 66, 69, 139–40
Brain disorders, 23, 74, 94
Brain injury, 138, 196
Brain tumors, 20–21, 23, 132
Brain wave recordings (EEG), 23, 147
Breast cancer, 60, 63, 96, 133–35, 186
Bronchitis, 19, 121, 143
  chronic, 95–96, 116, 180–81
Bronchoscopy, 19, 66, 72
Bulimia, 174
Buspar, 94

Caffeine, 93, 143
Calcium, 155, 164, 166–67, 183
Calcium channel blockers, 92, 93
Calcium deficiency, 97–98, 167
Cancer(s), 20, 22, 67, 70, 84, 99, 122, 138, 178
  of colon, 161
  of esophagus, 140
  gynecologic, 21, 73
  obesity and, 169, 184
  physical exam for early detection of, 187
  smoking and, 181, 182
  surgery in treatment of, 129, 131, 133–35
  of uninary tract, 135
  see also Breast cancer; Lung cancer; Prostate cancer
Cannabis, 139, 142–43
Carafate, 93
Carbohydrates, 154, 160–62, 173
Carbon, 154, 156–57, 160
Cardiac catheterization, 71
Cardiologist, 7, 19
Cardiomyopathy, 141
Cardiopulmonary resuscitation, 17, 18
Cardiovascular disease, 19, 138, 167
Cardiovascular drugs, 92–93, 104
Cardiovascular surgery, 132
Cardiovascular system, 141
CAT scan, 21–22, 58, 63, 64, 72, 73, 74, 131, 132
Catastrophic insurance coverage, 30, 34
Cellulose, 160, 161
CHAMPUS, 29
Checkups, 18, 118, 185–87
  insurance coverage, 31, 35, 50, 51
Chemical dependency, 86, 137–52
Chemical imbalances, 116, 123
Chemicals, 77, 147

Chemotherapy, 20, 79, 99, 114, 134, 135
Chest X rays, 58, 60, 62, 71, 72
Cholesterol, 97, 156, 161, 183–84
  good/bad, 157–59
  screening tests for, 56, 186–87
Chloramphenicol, 76
Cholestyramine, 97
Cirrhosis of liver, 141, 181
Clinical psychologists, 24
Clinicians, nonphysician, 8
Cocaine, 138, 143–44, 147–48, 181
Codeine, 95
Coinsurance, 31–32, 34, 42, 50
Cold medications, 95
Colds, 98, 164
Collagen, 163–64
Colon, 67, 72, 129, 161
Colon cancer screening, 187
Colonoscopy, 60, 67
Consent, 112–13, 190–91, 192
  see also Informed consent
Consultation, 196
  see also Referrals
Cooper, Kevin, 182
Copayment, 31, 34, 42, 45, 50
Copper, 164, 167
Coronary angiography, 19, 71
Coronary artery bypass graft (CABG), 114, 127, 129, 132
Cortisone, 78, 85, 90, 95, 96, 117
Cost sharing (health insurance) 31–32, 34, 42, 50, 51
Costs
  of health insurance, 30–32, 34–35, 47, 50
  of malpractice cases, 198
  of medications, 100–4
  of tests, 57, 60
Costs of medical care, 3, 27, 201–2
  efforts to control, 26, 27–28, 33, 51
  health insurance and, 42, 44, 51
Cough medicines, 95
Crack, 138, 143, 145
Crile, George, 133–34
Critical care, 19
Cultures, 70–71, 72, 73, 74
Cure(s), 84, 106, 128–29
Cystoscopy, 67, 73

Death, 39, 181, 182
  addiction and, 143, 147
  alcohol and, 140, 141
  from surgery, 113, 115, 117, 119, 132
Decision making (medical), 16, 26
  about medications, 75–76
  patient's right in, 191

about surgery, 113–14
Decongestants, 90, 95
Deep vein thrombosis (DVT), 121–22
Denial, 124, 148
Denys, Jean Baptiste, of Montpellier, 111
Dependence(y), 124, 143, 145–47
  see also Chemical dependency
Dependency substances, 139–44
Depressants, 138–42
Depression, 94, 124, 144
Dermatology, 18
Dextromethorphan, 95
deVigo, Jean, 107
Diabetes, 2, 19, 61, 74, 82, 85, 97, 116, 129, 135, 140, 177, 180, 185
  and postoperative complications, 123
  and surgical risk, 117
  treatment of, 85
Diagnosis, 7, 18, 31, 70, 72, 78
  of addiction, 144
  and malpractice, 194
  medical tests in, 19, 54, 59, 60–61, 74, 131, 191
  pathologists and, 22
Diarrhea, 2, 70, 93, 116, 140, 169
Diet, 114, 159, 172, 173, 177, 183
  balanced, 153, 154
  and calcium absorption, 166–67
  fiber in, 161–62
  low fat, 158, 159
Dieting, 90, 143, 170, 174
Dietitions, registered (R.D.), 172, 173, 175, 176, 178
Digestion, 141, 155, 169
Digitalis, 2, 81, 92
Digoxin, 61
Diphtheria vaccine, 87, 99, 184
Disease, 2, 3, 106, 108
  addiction as, 145–47
  defined, 145
  germ theory of, 2, 108, 109
  humoral theory of, 106
  medications in control of, 84, 85
Diuretics, 61, 76, 90–91, 92, 116, 117, 169
Doctor(s), 5–25
  availability of, 5, 13–14, 36
  choice of, and health insurance, 32–33, 35–36, 37, 42
  HMOs, 33, 35–36, 40, 51
  Medicare/Medicaid participating, 46–47, 49
  with nutrition specialization, 175
  personality of, 5, 15–16
Doctor-patient relationship, 15–16, 43
  communication in, 3, 4, 15, 16, 197
  duty in, 189, 190–191

Index

HMOs and, 36–37, 39
placebo effect and, 89
DPT vaccine, 87
Drew, Charles, 112
Drug abuse, 94, 138, 145–47
Drug delivery systems, 103
Drug errors, 195
Drug patents, 101–2
Drug screening, 59, 61, 93
Drugs, 159, 181
  of abuse, 138–39
  anesthetic, 195
  cost factor and generics, 100–4
  new, 3, 101, 114–15
  see also Medications; Toxicity
DTs (delirium tremens), 140, 149
Duodenum, 67, 71–72

Eating habits, 154, 173, 177, 179
Echocardiogram, 58, 71
Einthoven, Willem, 65
Elderly, the, 44–48, 124
Electrical recordings, 65–66
Electrocardiogram (EKG), 58, 65–66, 71, 187
Electroencephalogram (EEG), 23, 66, 74
Electromyogram (EMG), 23, 66, 74
Elixir Sulfanilamide, 100
Ellwood, Paul, 27
Emergency(ies), 18, 191, 195–96
Emotional disorders, 123–25, 149
Emphysema, 19, 72, 116, 117, 121, 180, 181, 185
  medications for, 95–96
Endocrine glands, 19, 96
Endocrine medications, 96
Endocrine system, 68, 72–73, 92, 169
Endocrinology, 19, 21
Endoscopy, 66–67, 71–72, 129–30
Enzyme tests, 68, 72
Epilepsy, 23, 66, 74, 85, 93
Ergotamine, 93
Esophagus, 67, 71–72, 140
Estrogen, 96, 142, 167, 187
Ether, 110
Exercise, 159, 160, 177, 182–83
  and weight, 171, 172, 173, 183
Extracorporeal lithotripsy, 131
Eyes, 22, 135

Facchinetti, Neil J., 103
Family practitioner(s), 6, 14, 18, 21, 22
Fansidar, 87
Fat cell theory, 170–71
Fats, 154, 156–60, 173, 183
Fatty acids, 156, 157

Feces, analysis of, 69–70
Fee-for-service, 26–27, 28, 37
  in health insurance, 40–41, 51
Fees, 14, 30–31, 46–47, 49
Fetal alcohol syndrome, 138, 142
Fetus, 21, 25
Fiber (dietary), 160, 161–62, 183
Fiberoptic endoscopes, 66–67
Fluoride, 98
Food, 80, 178–79, 183
Food additives, 153, 177
Food sources of nutrients, 155, 161, 164, 165–69, 165t, 178

Gallbladder surgery, 127, 131–32
Gallstones, 64, 72, 129, 131–32
Gangrene, 85, 108, 181
Gastroenterology, 19, 67
Gastrointestinal disease, 71–72, 123, 177
Gastrointestinal drugs, 93
Gastrointestinal system, 131, 140
Generalists, 5–8, 18
Generic drugs, 100–4
Genetic factors, 139, 147, 158, 171–72
Glandular system, 141–42
Glaucoma, 85, 135
Glucose, 160
Glycogen, 160
Gonorrhea, 74, 84, 181–82
Gout, 19, 69, 79, 97
Group practice, 13, 18, 27, 37–38, 51
Group therapies, 24, 149
Gynecologic disease, 73–74
Gynecology, 15, 21, 142

Habituation, 86, 90, 94
Hallucinogens, 139, 143, 145
Halstead, William, 109, 133
Hangover(s), 140, 145
Harvey, William, 108, 111
Hashish, 142
Health, 3, 6, 174, 179
Health care expectations, 198–99
Health insurance, 3, 5, 26–53
  basic benefits, 30, 34
  benefits and costs, 30–32
  capitation fee, 33, 37
  conventional, 29–33, 51, 52–53t
  deductible in, 31, 34, 45, 50
  forms of, 29
  history of, 26–29
  premium, 33, 35, 42, 50
  and quality of care, 38–41
  supplemental, 44, 45, 47–48
Health maintenance, 180–87

Health Maintenance organizations (HMOs), 8, 27–28, 33–41, 42, 51
  benefits and costs, 34–35
  features of, 52–53t
  freedom of choice and style, 35–37
  group model and IPA, 37–38
  and Medicare, 47–48
  quality of care, 38–41, 50
  surgical rates, 35, 41, 127
Heart attack, 71, 85, 86, 122, 143–44, 158
  obesity and, 183
  smoking and, 180, 181
Heart disease, 92, 115, 169, 177, 178
  drugs in treatment of, 92–93
  fats/cholesterol in, 156, 158–60
  medical tests for, 71
  and surgical risk, 116, 117
Heart failure, 1, 122, 141, 185
Heart rhythm irregularities, 65–66, 92–93, 141
Heart transplant, 1, 25, 136
Hematology, 7, 20
Hemoglobin, 55, 155, 163, 167
Hepatitis, 61, 68, 74, 117, 144
  alcoholic, 140–41
  non-A, non-B, 126
  tests for, 57
Hepatitis vaccine, 99, 100
Hernia, 129, 131
Heroin, 138, 144, 147
Herpes, 91, 181–82
Hiatus hernia, 113, 114
High blood pressure. See Hypertension
Hip joint replacement, 121, 127, 132–33
Hippocrates, 106
Holmes, Oliver Wendell, 108, 109
Home health care, 45
Hormones, 3, 90, 96, 104, 136, 154
  blood concentrations of, 68, 73
Hospital(s), 8, 10–11, 32–33, 36, 43, 119–20
  emergency rooms, 14, 18, 196
Hospitalization, 32, 35, 44–45
Hydrogen, 64, 154, 156–57, 160
Hypercholesterolemia, 159, 169, 177
Hypertension, 60, 63, 82, 85, 168, 169, 177, 178, 180
  alcohol and, 141
  drugs in treatment of, 79, 90, 92, 94, 98, 101–2
  and surgical risk, 115, 116
Hysterosalpingogram, 73

Iatrogenic disease, 3
Ibuprofen, 95, 123
Imaging, 61–65, 73

Imipramine (Tofranil), 94
Immune defense mechanisms, 76–77, 143, 185
Immune globulins, 100
Immune system, 17, 96, 99, 141, 155
Immunizations, 2, 31, 34, 98–100, 184–85
  active, passive, 98–100
Impotence, 135, 142
Indomethacin, 123
Infection(s), 69, 70–71, 81, 122, 141
  antibiotics in treatment of, 84, 91
  blood tests with, 68
  from IV drug use, 144
  in joint replacement, 133
  pneumococcus, 185
  postoperative, 123
  prevention of, 117
  spread by surgeons, 108–9
  susceptibility to, 116
  vaginal, 73–74
  wound, 121
Infectious disease, 20
Infertility, 21, 73, 84, 96
Influenza vaccine, 99, 185
Informed consent, 191, 192–93
Injuries, 118, 131, 156, 182, 183
Insomnia, 86, 94
Insulin, 81, 85, 96, 97, 116, 182
Insurance, malpractice, 201–2
  see also Health insurance
Internists, 14, 18–20, 21
Intoxication, 148
IPA (Independent Practice Association) model, 37–38, 51
Iron, 97, 164, 166–68
IVP (intravenous pyelogram), 62–63, 73

Johnson, Vern, 148
Joints, 20, 67, 69, 130
Joint replacement, 132–33

Kaiser-Permanante Medical Groups, 28
Kidney(s), 25, 73, 80, 82, 156
  tests of, 62, 63
Kidney disease, 20, 69, 84, 123
Kidney failure, 85, 122–23, 177, 186
Kidney stones, 19, 25, 70, 85, 86, 97, 131
  surgery for, 135
Kidney transplantation, 136

Labavius, Andreas, 110–11
Landsteiner, Karl, 112
Laser surgery, 130, 132, 135
Lasers, 21–22, 131
Laxatives, 90–91, 93, 169

Index

Life-style, 180–84
Lincoln, Abraham, 189
Lipoproteins, 157
Lister, Joseph, 109
Lithium, 94, 98
Liver, 68, 72, 80, 82, 117, 126, 157
   alcohol and, 140–41, 142
Lower, Richard, 111
LSD, 143, 145
Lumbar puncture (spinal tap), 74
Lung cancer, 19, 58, 60, 66, 143, 180, 181
Lung scan, 58, 65, 72
Lungs, 19, 66, 69, 72, 116
Lymph glands, 134–35, 187

Magnesium, 98
Major medical benefits, 30, 34, 51
Malnutrition, 116, 140
Malpractice (medical), 188–202
   breach of duty in, 189, 191–93
   causation in, 189, 193
   damages in, 189, 193–94, 197–98, 201–2
   defined, 189
   elements in, 189–94
   insurance crisis and, 201–2
Malpractice cases, 1, 18, 112, 196–201
   appeals in, 200
   costs in, 198
   out-of-court settlement of, 198, 201
   types of, 194–96
   validity of, 199
Mammography, 31, 34, 49, 63, 185, 186
Marijuana, 138, 142–43, 145, 181
Mastectomy, 133–35
Maternal and fetal medicine, 21
Measles and mumps vaccine (MMR), 184, 185
Measles vaccine, 87, 99, 184–85
Medicaid, 27, 28–29, 48–49
Medical boards, 17–25
Medical care, 60
   managed, 41–42, 51
Medical education, 1–2, 3–4, 5–6, 16, 18
Medical history, 29, 118, 186
Medical measurements, 54–56
Medical practice, 1, 26, 39
   see also Practice style
Medical services, 48–50
Medical tests, 14, 54–74
   accuracy of, 60
   commonly used, 61–71
   disorders and solutions, 71–74
   interpretation of, 56–57, 61, 74
   propose of, 59–61
Medicare, 9, 27, 28–29, 44–48

Medication history, 115, 117
Medications, 2, 49, 50, 74, 75–104, 132
   as alternative to surgery, 114–115, 127
   benefits of, 84–91
   blood levels of, 69, 80, 81–82, 83
   causing kidney failure, 122–23
   commonly used, 91–100
   costs of, 104
   delivery systems, 80
   dosage, 79–80, 81–83
   and emergency surgery, 118
   and metabolism, 96–98
   interactions of, 82–83
   for own sake, 84, 90–91
   and potassium retention, 169
   risks of, 76–83, 94
   see also Toxicity
Medicine, 1, 2, 3–4, 27, 105–6
   defensive, 201
   modern, 54, 189
Meningitis, 20, 23, 69, 74, 185
Menstruation, 73, 142
Metabolism, 19, 96–98, 170, 171
Microbes, 108, 109, 121
Microsurgery, 21–22, 131
Migraine, 93
Mineral supplements, 162–63, 173
Minerals, 97–98, 154, 166–69
Monotherapy, 93
Mood-altering drugs, 138–39
Morton, William T. G., 110
Motility disorders, 93
MRI (Magnetic Resonance Imaging), 24, 63–64, 73, 74
Multiple sclerosis, 23, 59, 69
Muscles, 23, 69, 74

Naranon, 151, 152
Narcotics, 78–79, 95, 139, 144, 145, 195
Narcotics Anonymous, 149
Negligence (legal theory), 189, 195, 196, 200, 202
   proving, 191–92, 193, 194
Nephrology, 7, 20
Nephrotomogram, 62
Neurologic drugs, 93–94
Neurology, 22, 23–24, 66
Neuromuscular disease, 74
Neuro-opthalmology, 22
Neuro/psychiatric disorders, 123–25
Neurosurgery, 13, 20–21, 132
Neurotransmitters, 147
Nervous system, 92, 142, 163
Nicotine, 138, 143, 181
Nitroglycerin, 80, 92

Nitrous oxide, 109–10
Nonsteroidal anti-inflammatory
    (NSAIDS) drugs, 95, 123
Normal (the) (defined), 54–56
Nuclear scans, 65
Nurse practitioners, 8
Nutrient supplements, 162–63, 165
Nutrients, 140, 153
    categories of, 154–69
Nutrition, 115, 153–79, 183
    and weight control, 172, 173
    vitamins and, 165–66
Nutrition management, 177, 178
Nutritionists, 175–78

Obesity, 159, 169–75, 176, 177, 183–84
    causes of, 169–70, 174
    defined, 169
    and surgical risk, 117, 121, 122
Obstetrics, 21, 40, 41, 49, 108–9
Oncology, 20, 21
Open-heart surgery, 13, 120, 124, 130
Ophthalmologists, 21–23
Orthopedic surgery, 132–33
Orthopedists, 22
Osler, William, 3
Osteoporosis, 98, 166, 167, 182, 187
Otolaryngology, 22
Outcomes, 9, 39, 40–41
    bad, 196, 198–99
Outpatient care, 31, 35, 44
Outpatient surgery, 131, 133
Ovaries, 19, 64, 68, 96, 187
Overdose, 139, 144
Oxygen, 154, 157, 160

Packed red blood cells (PRBC), 125
Pain, 108, 109–10, 124
Painkillers, 85–86, 93, 95, 124, 144
    habituation/addiction to, 90, 95
Pancreas, 68, 72, 73, 96
Pancreatitis, 140
PAP smear, 58, 70, 73, 184, 185, 186
    health insurance coverage, 31, 34, 49
Paré, Ambrose, 107–8
Pasteur, Louis, 108, 109
Pathologists, 22
Patient(s), 2–4, 191, 194
Pediatricians, 22–23
Penicillin, 77, 78, 81, 91
Precutaneous transluminal coronary angio-
    plasty (PTCA), 130
Pernicious anemia, 85, 163
Pharmaceutical industry, 100–1
Pharmacist(s), 82

Pharmacogenetics, 78
Pharmacokinetics, 79–80
Phenobarbital, 93
Phenothiazines, 94
Phenylbutazone (Butazolidin), 76
Phenytoin, 93
Phosphorus, 164, 166
Physical exam, 185–87
    and health insurance, 31, 47, 49
    see also Checkups
Physician's assistants (PAs), 8
Phytate, 167
Pituitary gland, 19, 68, 73, 96
Placebo, 84, 88–90
Plasma, 112, 125
Plastic surgery, 23, 124
Pleural fluid analysis, 69
Pneumococcal disease, 185
Pneumococcal pneumonia vaccine, 99
Pneumonia, 19, 84, 116, 121, 185
Polio vaccine, 87, 99
Polysaccharides, 160, 161
Poor (the), 16, 26, 28–29, 39
Postoperative complications, 20, 120–26
Potassium, 55, 61, 81, 168–69
Potassium deficiency, 97, 116, 123, 169
Practice style, 5, 15–16, 36, 43, 51
Preferred Provider Organization (PPO), 28,
    41–43, 50, 51–52
    features of, 52–53t
Pregnancy, 21, 49, 84, 87–88, 98, 156, 164,
    165, 168, 177, 180, 184
alcohol use during, 142
calcium needs in, 166–67
complications of, 181
tests for, 56
Prevention
    atherosclerosis, 159–60
    deep vein thrombosis, 122
    immunizations in, 99, 184
    medications in, 84, 86–88, 93
    of need for emergency surgery, 118
    surgery in, 129
Preventive medicine, 3, 18, 23, 182
    annual physical in, 185, 186
    and health insurance, 31, 34, 49, 50, 51
Primary care physician, 6–7, 14, 17, 18, 36,
    37
    health insurance and, 42
    internist as, 18
    referrals by, 19, 21, 42–43, 51
Probenecid, 97
Prophylactic surgery, 129, 132
PROs (Peer Review Organizations), 9
Prostate cancer, 96

Index

Prostate gland, 25, 64, 68, 73, 135, 187
Prostheses, 23, 25
Proteins, 116, 141, 154–56, 166, 173
  in urine, 73
Psychiatric nurses, 24
Psychiatric conditions, 191, 196
Psychiatry, 23–24
Psychoactive drugs, 94, 124
Psychoanalysis, 23–24
Psychological factors in obesity, 169, 174, 183
Psychosis, 143
Psychotherapy, 23, 24
Public health, 23, 59, 60
Puerperal fever, 108–9
Pulmonary disease, 19, 169
Pulmonary function tests, 72
Pyridoxine, 163

Quality of care, 38–41, 50–51
Quality of life, 113–14

Rabies vaccine, 86, 99, 100
Radiation, 21, 63, 114, 134, 135, 136
Radioactive imagings, 64–65
Radioactive materials, 25, 64–65, 71
Radioactive scans, 72, 73
Radioimmunoassays, 68, 73
Radiology, 24–25, 61–65
Rare diseases, testing for, 59–60
Rectum, 72
Referrals, 8, 19, 21, 23, 36, 42–43
  health insurance and, 43, 51
Rejection phenomenon, 136
Respiratory medications, 95–96
Retrovir, 91, 101
Rheumatoid arthritis, 17, 85, 169
Rheumatology, 20
Risk(s)
  of medications, 76–83
  surgical, 115–20, 195
  in tests, 57–58
Risks/benefits
  of medications, 75–76, 85, 86, 87, 88, 89
  in surgery, 112–15, 127
  in tests, 57–58, 62
Rubella immunization, 99, 184
Rush, Benjamin, 2

Screening tests, 6, 31, 59, 60
Scientific method, 1, 107
Second opinion(s), 91, 127–28
Sedatives, 94, 98
Semmelweis, Agnaz Philipp, 108–9
Set-point theory, 171

Sexually transmitted diseases, 59, 74, 181–82
SGOT, 61
Shock, 108,, 122
Shock wave therapy, 25, 131, 132
Side effects, 92, 94, 95, 96, 114, 163
Sigmoidoscopy, 66, 67
Skilled nursing facilities, 45
Skin disorders, 17–18
Sleeping pills, 90, 94, 139
Sleep-apnea syndrome, 22
SMA, 12, 68
Smallpox, 1, 86–87, 99
Smith, David, 145
Smoking, 115, 132, 159, 180–81, 183
  and surgical risk, 116, 117, 121
Social workers, 24
Sodium, 55, 97, 168, 183
Sonogram, 24–25, 73
Specialists, 5–8, 36, 190, 196
Specialties, 17–25
Sperm count, 69
Spleen, 141, 185
Spinal cord, 20–21, 23, 69, 74
Spinal fluid, 69, 74
Spinal tap, 74
Spirometry, 72
Sports medicine, 22, 23
Sputum, 70, 72
Standard of care, 190, 193, 199
  and breach of duty, 191–92
Sterilization, 109, 130
Stimulants, 90, 139, 143–44
Stomach, 67, 71–72, 140
Stomach acid, 69, 93
Stool, blood in, 60, 72, 187
Streptococci, 70
Streptomycin, 91
Stress test, 19, 71
Stroke, 2, 63, 74, 85, 143, 158, 181, 186
Subspecialties, 6, 7, 18–20, 42–43, 196
  gynecology, 21
  pediatrics, 22–23
  radiology, 25
Substance abuse, 137–52
Sucralfate, 84
Sugar, 161
Suicide, 138, 144
Sulfanilamide, 100
Surgeon(s), 7, 12–13, 14, 19, 21, 22, 25, 127
Surgery, 2, 18, 22, 66, 105–36
  alternatives to, 114–15, 127
  colon/rectal, 17
  complications with, 120–26
  conditions requiring, 115–16
  elective, 117–18

emergency, 117–19, 121, 128
gynecologic, 142
health insurance and frequency of, 35, 41, 127
history of, 105–12
kinds of, 131–36
and malpractice, 192, 195
modern, 112, 136
obesity and, 184
reconstructive, restorative, 129
risk-benefit ratio in, 112–15, 127, 128–29
risks of, 115–28
spread of infection in, 108–9
unnecessary, 126–28
Surgical techniques, 129–31, 136
Symptoms, 84, 85–86, 146
Syphilis, 56, 74, 181–82

Tagamet, 93
Technology, 2–3, 7, 19, 21–22
Testicles, 19, 68, 96, 142, 187
Testosterone, 96
Tetanus vaccine, 99, 100, 184
Theophylline preparations, 80, 95
Thyroid gland, 19, 57, 65, 68, 73, 117, 187
Thyroid deficiency, 84–85, 96
Tolerance, 95, 146, 147
Tomogram, 62
Toxicity, 20, 61, 81, 94, 100, 104, 124, 136
chemical, 78–79
minerals, 98
nutrient supplements, 163
potassium, 169
vitamins, 163
Tranquilizers, 79, 90, 94, 138, 139
Transdermal delivery systems, 80
Transplantation surgery, 1, 17, 25, 135–36
Transurethral surgery, 135
Treatment, 74
of addiction, 148–50, 152
availability of tests and, 59–60
inappropriate, 191
and malpractice, 191, 192
placebo effect of, 89

questions about, 196–97
Treatment errors, 195
Tumors, 67, 72, 73, 74
Twelve Step Programs, 149–50, 151, 152

Uclers, 67, 69, 84, 86, 93, 130, 181
Ultrasound, 21–22, 64, 72, 73, 135
in surgery, 131
Upper GI series, 62
Uric acid, 69, 97
Urinary tract disease, 73
Urine analysis, 69, 70, 123
Urologic surgery, 135
Urologist, 7, 25, 64

Vaccines, 6, 68, 75–76, 86–87, 99–100, 184
Valium, 90, 94, 140
Vascular anastomosis, 136
Vasodilators, 92
Vegetarianism, 155, 177
Vertigo, 94
Vesalius, Andreas, 107, 108
Viral infections, 144
Viruses, 20, 70, 91
Vitamin deficiency, 98, 142, 162, 164, 165
Vitamin supplements, 154, 162–63, 173
Vitamins, 85, 98, 154, 157, 162–66, 183
Vomiting, 94, 116, 118, 140, 169

Waller, Augustus, 65
Warren, John C., 110
Washington, George, 2
Water, 154, 169
Weight, 169, 171, 172–73, 174, 178
Weight control program, 172–74
Weight loss, 175–76, 183
Wells, Horace, 110
White blood cells, 68, 73, 141, 167
Withdrawal reaction(s), 139, 140, 144, 145, 147

X rays, 24–25, 62, 63, 64

Zantac, 93
Zinc, 98, 155, 167